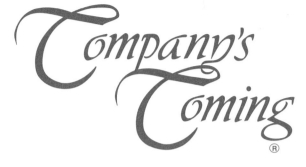

Healthy Recipe Makeovers

Jean Paré

www.companyscoming.com
visit our website

Front Cover

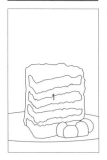

1. Mocha Layer Cake,
   page 150

Back Cover

1. FLT Tacos, page 73
2. Simply Fresh Salsa,
   page 120
3. Veggie Bean
   Enchiladas, page 94
4. Salsa Beef Tacos,
   page 34

Props:
Moderno

Healthy Recipe Makeovers

Copyright © Company's Coming Publishing Limited

First Printing January 2012

Library and Archives Canada Cataloguing in Publication
Paré, Jean, date
Healthy recipe makeovers / Jean Paré.
(Original series)
Includes index.
At head of title: Company's coming.
ISBN 978-1-897477-78-6
1. Cooking. 2. Cookbooks. I. Title. II. Series: Paré, Jean, date. Original series.
TX714.P3565 2012   641.5   C2011-904323-8

We gratefully acknowledge the following suppliers for their generous support of our Test and Photography Kitchens:

Broil King Barbecues
Corelle®
Hamilton Beach® Canada
Lagostina®
Proctor Silex® Canada
Tupperware®

Published by
Company's Coming Publishing Limited
2311 – 96 Street
Edmonton, Alberta, Canada T6N 1G3
Tel: 780-450-6223   Fax: 780-450-1857
www.companyscoming.com

We acknowledge the financial support of the Government of Canada through the Canada Book Fund for our publishing activities.

Printed in China

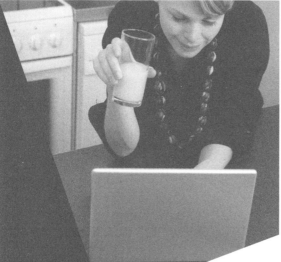
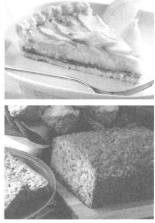

Company's Coming Cookbooks

Continue down the path to a healthier lifestyle!
Try some of our other healthy titles.

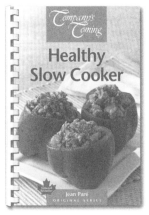

Original Series

- Softcover, 160 pages
- Lay-flat plastic comb binding
- Full-colour photos
- Nutrition information

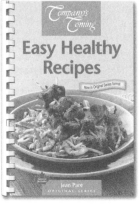

Original Series

- Softcover, 160 pages
- Lay-flat plastic comb binding
- Full-colour photos
- Nutrition information

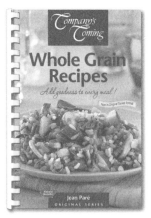

Original Series

- Softcover, 160 pages
- Lay-flat plastic comb binding
- Full-colour photos
- Nutrition information

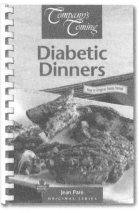

Original Series

- Softcover, 160 pages
- Lay-flat plastic comb binding
- Full-colour photos
- Nutrition information

For a complete listing of our cookbooks, visit our website:
www.companyscoming.com

Table of Contents

Makeover the
Way You Eat

Salads & Soups

Beef

Fish & Seafood

Vegetarian

Sides

Baking

Desserts

The Company's Coming Story

Jean Paré (pronounced "jeen PAIR-ee") grew up understanding that the combination of family, friends and home cooking is the best recipe for a good life. From her mother, she learned to appreciate good cooking, while her father praised even her earliest attempts in the kitchen. When Jean left home, she took with her a love of cooking, many family recipes and an intriguing desire to read cookbooks as if they were novels!

"Never share a recipe you wouldn't use yourself."

When her four children had all reached school age, Jean volunteered to cater the 50th anniversary celebration of the Vermilion School of Agriculture, now Lakeland College, in Alberta, Canada. Working out of her home, Jean prepared a dinner for more than 1,000 people, launching a flourishing catering operation that continued for over 18 years. During that time, she had countless opportunities to test new ideas with immediate feedback—resulting in empty plates and contented customers! Whether preparing cocktail sandwiches for a house party or serving a hot meal for 1,500 people, Jean Paré earned a reputation for great food, courteous service and reasonable prices.

As requests for her recipes increased, Jean was often asked the question, "Why don't you write a cookbook?" Jean responded by teaming up with her son, Grant Lovig, in the fall of 1980 to form Company's Coming Publishing Limited. The publication of *150 Delicious Squares* on April 14, 1981 marked the debut of what would soon become one of the world's most popular cookbook series.

The company has grown since those early days when Jean worked from a spare bedroom in her home. Today, she continues to write recipes while working closely with the staff of the Recipe Factory, as the Company's Coming test kitchen is affectionately known. There she fills the role of mentor, assisting with the development of recipes people most want to use for everyday cooking and easy entertaining. Every Company's Coming recipe is *kitchen-tested* before it is approved for publication.

Company's Coming cookbooks are distributed in Canada, the United States, Australia and other world markets. Bestsellers many times over in English, Company's Coming cookbooks have also been published in French and Spanish.

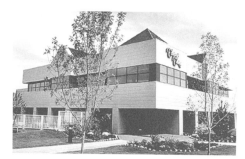

Familiar and trusted in home kitchens around the world, Company's Coming cookbooks are offered in a variety of formats. Highly regarded as kitchen workbooks, the softcover Original Series, with its lay-flat plastic comb binding, is still a favourite among readers.

Jean Paré's approach to cooking has always called for *quick and easy recipes* using *everyday ingredients*. That view has served her well. The recipient of many awards, including the Queen Elizabeth Golden Jubilee Medal, Jean was appointed Member of the Order of Canada, her country's highest lifetime achievement honour.

Jean continues to gain new supporters by adhering to what she calls The Golden Rule of Cooking: *Never share a recipe you wouldn't use yourself.* It's an approach that has worked—*millions of times over!*

Foreword

These days, most of us want to eat healthier. But even though we have the best intentions, we keep going back to the same old foods. Wouldn't it be great if there were a way to enjoy our favourite foods and eat healthily at the same time?

There is—with *Healthy Recipe Makeovers*! In this book, we've taken some of your favourite recipes and spruced them up with fresh new makeovers. These remakes are not only every bit as good as the originals, but they're good for you as well!

How does a recipe get a makeover? We've chosen naturally healthier ingredients such as whole grains and leaner cuts of meat. We've upped the nutritional content wherever we can, adding fibre and packing recipes full of nutrient-rich fruits and veggies. We've used healthier cooking methods, like roasting in the oven instead of deep-frying. And we've cut back on ingredients that are high in calories, fat and sodium, using small amounts only when it's absolutely necessary.

Many people's favourite foods fall into the category of comfort food—those warm, comforting dishes that conjure up childhood memories and never fail to make you feel good. Often we see comfort food and other "guilty pleasures" as unhealthy indulgences. There's no need to give up these comforts entirely! Comfort and indulgence foods are the dishes most in need of healthy makeovers, and that's exactly what we've done.

You'll find a wide range of recipes in this book, from appetizers and main dishes to sides and desserts—and even condiments and sauces. The amazingly low-fat Spinach Dip will get rave reviews from your friends, and our update of the classic Cordon Bleu Chicken is simply to die for. You'll also discover new favourites, like the unique Pepper Quinoa Pizza. Then top off your meal with delicious, fruit-filled Cherry Almond Crepes.

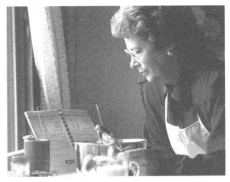

You can absolutely enjoy your favourite foods without feeling guilty. Let *Healthy Recipe Makeovers* change the way you eat!

Jean Paré

Nutrition Information Guidelines

Each recipe is analyzed using the most current versions of the Canadian Nutrient File from Health Canada, and the United States Department of Agriculture (USDA) Nutrient Database for Standard Reference.

- If more than one ingredient is listed (such as "butter or hard margarine"), or if a range is given (1 – 2 tsp., 5 – 10 mL), only the first ingredient or first amount is analyzed.
- For meat, poultry and fish, the recommended serving size per person is 4 oz. (113 g) uncooked weight (without bone), which is 2 – 3 oz. (57 – 85 g) cooked weight (without bone)—approximately the size of a deck of playing cards.
- Milk used is 1% M.F. (milk fat), unless otherwise stated.
- Cooking oil used is canola oil, unless otherwise stated.
- Ingredients indicating "sprinkle," "optional" or "for garnish" are not included in the nutrition information.
- The fat in recipes and combination foods can vary greatly depending upon the sources and types of fats used in each specific ingredient. For these reasons, the amount of saturated, monounsaturated and polyunsaturated fats may not add up to the total fat content.

Makeover the Way You Eat

It *is* possible to eat healthier! The decision to eat better is a lifestyle choice that everyone can make, but it usually doesn't happen overnight. It starts with eliminating "bad habit" foods that have little or no nutritional value, and gradually adding in healthier options for meals and snacks. You can enjoy a healthier, more balanced diet without sacrificing the convenience factor of some less-nutritious foods—all it takes is a little planning and commitment.

Planning Ahead

Planning your meals ahead of time is a great way to help you stick to your nutrition goals without resorting to convenience or fast foods. Make a weekly meal plan and create your shopping list accordingly—it will make your trips to the grocery store or market so much more efficient. Planning and creating lists might seem like a lot of work, but the time you save overall justifies the extra effort. Putting together a balanced meal in the evening is a breeze if you know what you're making ahead of time—no more last-minute scrambling and hunting through your pantry!

Another time-saving idea is to get any prep work for your planned meal done the night before. For example, take meat out of the freezer the night before and let it thaw in the fridge. You won't be tempted to opt for takeout when you know you have something waiting to be cooked up—and you won't encounter those rubbery edges that mysteriously appear when you defrost meat in the microwave.

You can also double or triple a recipe and freeze the extras in meal-sized portions—that way you'll have ready-made meals to pack for lunches or to pull out for dinner on busy nights! Ensure that food is completely cooled before storing in airtight containers, and label the containers with the date and contents before putting them in the freezer.

Tips for Healthy Eating

Take small steps toward a positive lifestyle change! It's a good idea to reduce the overall fat, sodium and sugar that you consume. Including more whole grains in your overall diet is a great method for increasing your fibre intake: try barley, brown rice, oats, quinoa and wild rice.

Focus on using fresh ingredients instead of convenience products, which often include large amounts of fat, sodium and sugar. Try to eat fruit and vegetables every day, and choose dark green and orange vegetables more often—they contain the most vitamins and antioxidants. Here's a time-saving trick: frozen vegetables are almost always just as nutritious as fresh ones, so keep a supply of frozen veggies in the freezer that you can whip up in a hurry if you run out of fresh vegetables.

Trim all fat from meat and remove the skin from poultry, and drain away any fat that accumulates while cooking. Regularly include meat alternatives such as beans, lentils and tofu in your diet, and eat a few servings of fish each week.

Have a couple servings of dairy products such as milk, cheese or yogurt every day to get vitamin D. Look for lower-fat products in this category.

Enhance the flavour of dishes using fresh herbs, salt-free seasonings, spices or vinegars instead of adding extra salt.

Don't forget to read food labels! Learn what ingredients were used in the food you eat—remember, what goes into your food also goes into your body. You can also refer to *Canada's Food Guide* for general tips about food groups and portion sizes.

In This Book

You'll notice that we've followed our own advice for healthy eating with the recipe makeovers in this book! We focused on using fresh and natural ingredients: fresh and frozen vegetables, whole grains, lean cuts of meat and other natural foods. We also used healthy fats, such as canola oil and olive oil. Since butter is a natural food that lends its distinct flavour to the food it's cooked with, we also choose to include a few recipes that call for small amounts.

You may notice that the recipes in *Healthy Recipe Makeovers* use a couple of variations on the same ingredient. For example, in some spots we have opted for low-sodium broths, and in other recipes we have used regular. For the most part we've made limited use of "light" or non- or low-fat ingredients. We wanted to make sure that the recipes in *Healthy Recipe Makeovers* still taste great, too! Of course, it's up to you whether you wish to substitute for lighter products in these recipes. Keep in mind that when using lighter products, a dash of extra salt or seasoning may be required to pump up the flavour. And if you choose to make substitutions, remember that low-fat products often have a different consistency, which may affect the end result.

We evaluated nutritional information very carefully when creating *Healthy Recipe Makeovers*. Recipe makeovers had to not only meet the usual Company's Coming standards for excellence, but also had to be lower in calories, lower in fat and lower in sodium. In this book, *low fat* means under 10 g per serving, *low sodium* refers to recipes with under 140 mg per serving and *high fibre* indicates more than 3 g per serving.

Snappy Snack Bars

These sweet, nut-free bars are great for school lunches. Store at room temperature, or place wrapped bars in a resealable freezer bag to freeze for longer storage. To make them gluten-free, use gluten-free oats and cereal.

Large flake rolled oats	2 cups	500 mL
Flaked coconut	1 cup	250 mL
Unsalted raw sunflower seeds	1 cup	250 mL
Can of low-fat sweetened condensed milk	11 oz.	300 mL
Butter, melted	2 tbsp.	30 mL
Liquid honey	2 tbsp.	30 mL
Salt	1/2 tsp.	2 mL
Cooked quinoa (3/4 cup, 175 mL, uncooked)	2 cups	500 mL
Crisp rice cereal	2 cups	500 mL
Chopped dried apricot	1 1/2 cups	375 mL
Dried cranberries	1 cup	250 mL

BEFORE: *1 bar:*
203 Calories; 6 g Total Fat (3 g Sat); **210 g Sodium**

AFTER: *1 bar:*
139 Calories; 4.5 g Total Fat (0.5 g Mono, 1.5 g Poly, 1.5 g Sat); 3 mg Cholesterol; 22 g Carbohydrate; 2 g Fibre; 3 g Protein; **70 mg Sodium**

Line 10 x 15 inch (25 x 38 cm) baking sheet with sides with parchment paper, leaving 1 inch (2.5 cm) overhang on long sides. Set aside. Spread first 3 ingredients on ungreased baking sheet with sides. Bake in 350°F (175°C) oven for about 10 minutes, stirring every 5 minutes, until coconut is golden.

Whisk next 4 ingredients in large bowl.

Add remaining 4 ingredients and rolled oat mixture. Stir well. Press firmly into prepared pan. Bake in 325°F (160°C) oven for about 35 minutes until set and golden. Run knife along inside edge of pan to loosen. Let stand in pan on wire rack until cooled completely. Remove from pan. Cut lengthwise into thirds. Cut each third into 12 bars. Wrap bars individually in plastic wrap. Makes 36 bars.

Paré Pointer

The woman covered herself with vanishing cream.
No one knows where she went.

Spicy Sausage Rolls

After baking, rolls can be frozen for up to one month. Reheat from frozen in a 375ºF (190ºC) oven for about 12 minutes until heated through.

Canola oil	2 tsp.	10 mL
Chopped onion	2 cups	500 mL
Finely chopped fennel bulb (white part only)	2 cups	500 mL
Dried crushed chilies	2 tsp.	10 mL
Dried oregano	1 tsp.	5 mL
Dried thyme	1 tsp.	5 mL
Finely chopped peeled tart apple (such as Granny Smith)	1 1/2 cups	375 mL
Large flake rolled oats	1/3 cup	75 mL
Salt	1/2 tsp.	2 mL
Pepper	1/4 tsp.	1 mL
Lean ground turkey thigh	1/2 lb.	225 g
Phyllo pastry sheets, thawed according to package directions	4	4
Cooking spray		

BEFORE: *1 roll:*
162 Calories; *11 g Total Fat (2.6 Sat); 259 mg Sodium*

AFTER: *1 roll:*
20 Calories; *0.5 g Total Fat (0 g Mono, 0 g Poly, 0 g Sat); 3 mg Cholesterol; 3 g Carbohydrate; 0 g Fibre; 1 g Protein; 43 mg Sodium*

Heat canola oil in large frying pan on medium. Add next 5 ingredients. Cook for about 12 minutes, stirring often, until onion and fennel are softened.

Add apple. Stir. Cook for about 8 minutes until fennel is very soft. Remove from heat. Let stand for 20 minutes, stirring occasionally.

Combine next 3 ingredients in large bowl. Add apple mixture. Stir. Add turkey. Mix well.

Spray 1 pastry sheet with cooking spray. Place another one over top. Spray with cooking spray. Repeat, layering remaining pastry sheets and spraying with cooking spray. Cut pastry stack crosswise into 4 rectangles. Divide turkey mixture into 4 portions. Shape 1 portion on sheet of waxed paper into 13 inch (33 cm) long log. Transfer to long side of 1 pastry rectangle. Brush opposite long edge with water. Roll to enclose filling. Press seam against roll to seal. Repeat with remaining turkey mixture and pastry rectangles for a total of 4 rolls. Spray rolls with cooking spray. Cut each roll into 12 pieces. Using sharp knife, cut small slash across top of each piece. Arrange, seam-side down, on greased baking sheet with sides. Bake in 400ºF (205ºC) oven for about 20 minutes until pastry is golden and turkey is no longer pink inside. Makes 48 rolls.

Lemon Sesame Hummus

Lower in fat and calories than traditional hummus. The lovely light texture is layered with flavours of lemon, toasted sesame and a touch of chili heat.

Can of chickpeas (garbanzo beans), rinsed and drained	19 oz.	540 mL
Water	1/4 cup	60 mL
Lemon juice	3 tbsp.	50 mL
Roasted sesame seeds	3 tbsp.	50 mL
Olive oil	1 tbsp.	15 mL
Chopped fresh hot chili pepper (see Tip, page 13)	1/2 tsp.	2 mL
Garlic clove, chopped (or 1/4 tsp., 1 mL, powder)	1	1
Grated lemon zest (see Tip, page 151)	1/4 tsp.	1 mL
Salt	1/4 tsp.	1 mL
Chopped fresh parsley	2 tbsp.	30 mL

Process first 9 ingredients in food processor until smooth. Transfer to serving bowl.

Stir in parsley. Makes about 1 3/4 cups (425 mL).

BEFORE: *1/4 cup (60 mL): 164 Calories; **12.4 g Total Fat** (1.6 g Sat); 147 mg Sodium*

AFTER: *1/4 cup (60 mL): 70 Calories; **4 g Total Fat** (2 g Mono, 1 g Poly, 0.5 g Sat); 0 mg Cholesterol; 9 g Carbohydrate; 3 g Fibre; 3 g Protein; 167 mg Sodium*

Salt and Pepper Edamame

Instead of reaching for that nut mix, why not try roasted soybeans? They have just the right amount of crunch and make a great healthy snack.

Sesame oil (for flavour)	1 tbsp.	15 mL
Onion powder	1 tsp.	5 mL
Salt	1 tsp.	5 mL
Pepper	1/2 tsp.	2 mL
Garlic powder	1/2 tsp.	2 mL
Frozen shelled edamame (soybeans), thawed and blotted dry	4 cups	1 L

(continued on next page)

Stir first 5 ingredients in large bowl.

Add edamame. Stir to coat. Spread on greased baking sheet with sides. Bake in 350°F (175°C) oven for about 1 hour, stirring occasionally, until browned and crisp. Let stand until cool. Makes about 1 3/4 cups (425 mL).

BEFORE: *1/4 cup (60 mL): 216 Calories;* **17.8 g Total Fat** *(2.7 g Sat); 161 mg Sodium*

AFTER: *1/4 cup (60 mL): 120 Calories;* **5 g Total Fat** *(1 g Mono, 1 g Poly, 0 g Sat); 0 mg Cholesterol; 11 g Carbohydrate; 3 g Fibre; 8 g Protein; 340 mg Sodium*

Cheddar Chili Tarts

Whole-wheat flour tortillas are a great low-fat alternative to pastry in these tasty tarts.

Whole-wheat flour tortillas (10 inch, 25 cm, diameter)	4	4
Grated sharp Cheddar cheese	1/2 cup	125 mL
Large eggs	2	2
Milk	1/2 cup	125 mL
Dried crushed chilies	1/2 tsp.	2 mL
Pepper	1/4 tsp.	1 mL

Cut twelve 4 inch (10 cm) rounds from tortillas. Press rounds into greased muffin cups. Bake in 400°F (205°C) oven for about 8 minutes until golden and crisp. Let stand for 15 minutes. Reduce heat to 350°F (175°C).

Scatter cheese into tortilla cups.

Whisk remaining 4 ingredients in small bowl. Pour over cheese. Bake for about 20 minutes until puffed and set. Makes 12 tarts.

Pictured on page 17.

BEFORE: *1 tart:* **179 Calories**; *12.9 g Total Fat (6.6 g Sat); 179 mg Sodium*

AFTER: *1 tart:* **59 Calories**; *3 g Total Fat (1.5 g Mono, 0 g Poly, 1 g Sat); 25 mg Cholesterol; 5 g Carbohydrate; 1 g Fibre; 3 g Protein; 122 mg Sodium*

tip Hot peppers contain capsaicin in the seeds and ribs. Removing the seeds and ribs will reduce the heat. Wear rubber gloves when handling hot peppers and avoid touching your eyes. Wash your hands well afterwards.

Pepper Cheese Sticks

A great make-ahead appetizer. You can store baked cheese sticks in an airtight container in the freezer for up to one month. Reheat from frozen in a 375°F (190°C) oven for about 7 minutes until crisp and heated through.

Grated sharp Cheddar cheese	1 1/4 cups	300 mL
All-purpose flour	1 cup	250 mL
Whole-wheat flour	1 cup	250 mL
Coarsely ground pepper	1 tbsp.	15 mL
Salt	1/2 tsp.	2 mL
Cold butter, cut up	2/3 cup	150 mL
Cold water	1/2 cup	125 mL

BEFORE: *2 sticks:*
79 Calories; **6.6 g Total Fat** *(2.8 g Sat);*
66 mg Sodium

AFTER: *2 sticks:*
38 Calories; **2.5 g Total Fat** *(0.5 g Mono, 0 g Poly, 1.5 g Sat); 7 mg Cholesterol; 3 g Carbohydrate; 0 g Fibre; 1 g Protein; 43 mg Sodium*

Combine first 5 ingredients in large bowl. Cut in butter until mixture resembles coarse crumbs.

Slowly add water, stirring with fork, until mixture starts to come together. Do not overmix. Turn out dough onto work surface. Shape into flattened disc. Wrap with plastic wrap. Chill for 30 minutes. Divide dough into 2 equal portions. Roll out 1 portion on lightly floured surface into 10 x 16 inch (25 x 40 cm) rectangle. Cut in half lengthwise. Cut crosswise into 1/2 inch (12 mm) wide strips. Arrange on parchment paper-lined baking sheet with sides. Repeat with remaining dough. Bake in 400°F (205°C) oven for about 10 minutes until golden and crisp. Makes about 128 pastry sticks.

Paré Pointer

Heard about nitrates? They're supposed to be cheaper than day rates.

Blue Chicken Wings

Way better for you than the deep-fried restaurant variety! Chicken drumettes are the meatiest part of the chicken wing, so you get a better meat-to-fat ratio. This recipe also gives you a delicious homemade chicken stock. Simply chill the cooking liquid overnight, then remove and discard any fat before using.

Water	6 cups	1.5 L
Chicken drumettes	3 lbs.	1.4 kg
Medium carrots, quartered	2	2
Medium onion, quartered	1	1
Bay leaf	1	1
Apricot jam	1/4 cup	60 mL
Louisiana hot sauce	2 tbsp.	30 mL
Salt	1/4 tsp.	1 mL
LIGHT BLUE DIP		
95% fat-free spreadable cream cheese	1/4 cup	60 mL
Crumbled blue cheese	1/4 cup	60 mL
Light sour cream	1/4 cup	60 mL
Chopped chives (or green onion)	3 tbsp.	50 mL

BEFORE: *1 drumette and 1 tsp. (5 mL) dip:*
230 Calories; **18 g Total Fat** *(5 g Sat);*
430 mg Sodium

AFTER: *1 drumette and 1 tsp. (5 mL) dip:*
120 Calories; **8 g Total Fat** *(3 g Mono, 1.5 g Poly, 2.5 g Sat);*
39 mg Cholesterol;
2 g Carbohydrate;
0 g Fibre; 10 g Protein;
114 mg Sodium

Combine first 5 ingredients in Dutch oven or large pot. Bring to a boil. Reduce heat to medium. Simmer, uncovered, for about 20 minutes until drumettes are no longer pink inside. Strain cooking liquid into medium bowl. Reserve for another use. Remove and discard carrot, onion and bay leaf.

Stir next 3 ingredients in large bowl. Add hot drumettes. Toss until jam is melted and drumettes are coated. Transfer to greased foil-lined baking sheet with sides, reserving apricot mixture in bowl. Bake in 450°F (230°C) oven for about 20 minutes, turning occasionally, until browned. Toss drumettes in remaining apricot mixture. Makes about 28 chicken wings.

Light Blue Dip: Combine all 4 ingredients in small bowl. Makes about 2/3 cup (150 mL) dip. Serve with wings.

Pictured on page 17.

Baked Potato Skins

These nicely seasoned potato shells are loaded with flavour and healthier ingredients. Tasty, filling and crowd-pleasing.

Medium unpeeled baking potatoes	4	4
Canola oil	2 tbsp.	30 mL
Dry mustard	1/4 tsp.	1 mL
Garlic powder	1/4 tsp.	1 mL
Paprika	1/4 tsp.	1 mL
Salt	1/8 tsp.	0.5 mL
Pepper	1/4 tsp.	1 mL
Chopped deli smoked turkey slices	1/3 cup	75 mL
Chopped red pepper	1/4 cup	60 mL
Frozen tiny peas, thawed	1/4 cup	60 mL
Thinly sliced green onion	3 tbsp.	50 mL
Grated part-skim mozzarella cheese	1 cup	250 mL

Wrap each potato in foil. Bake directly on centre rack in 425°F (220°C) oven for about 1 1/2 hours until tender. Transfer to cutting board. Carefully remove foil. Let stand until cool enough to handle. Halve potatoes lengthwise. Scoop out pulp, leaving 1/4 inch (6 mm) shells. Reserve pulp for another use. Halve shells crosswise.

Combine next 6 ingredients in small cup. Brush over both sides of shells. Place shells, skin-side up, on ungreased baking sheet with sides. Bake for about 10 minutes until starting to brown. Turn shells over.

Combine next 4 ingredients in small bowl. Spoon into shells.

Sprinkle with cheese. Bake for about 5 minutes until cheese is melted. Makes 16 potato skins.

Pictured at right.

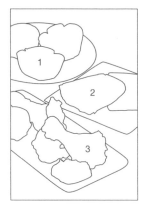

1. Cheddar Chili Tarts, page 13
2. Baked Potato Skins, above
3. Blue Chicken Wings, page 15

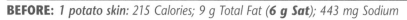

BEFORE: *1 potato skin: 215 Calories; 9 g Total Fat (6 g Sat); 443 mg Sodium*

AFTER: *1 potato skin: 80 Calories; 3 g Total Fat (1.5 g Mono, 0.5 g Poly, 1 g Sat); 4 mg Cholesterol; 12 g Carbohydrate; 1 g Fibre; 3 g Protein; 80 mg Sodium*

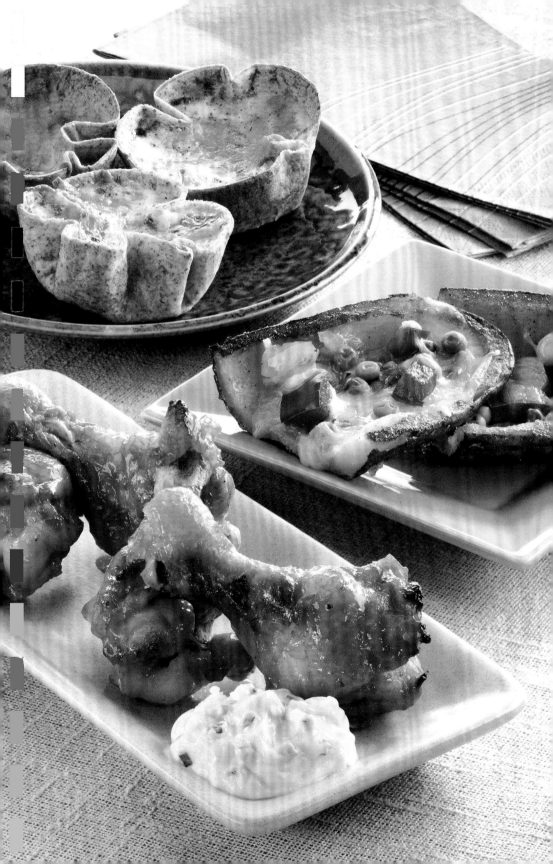

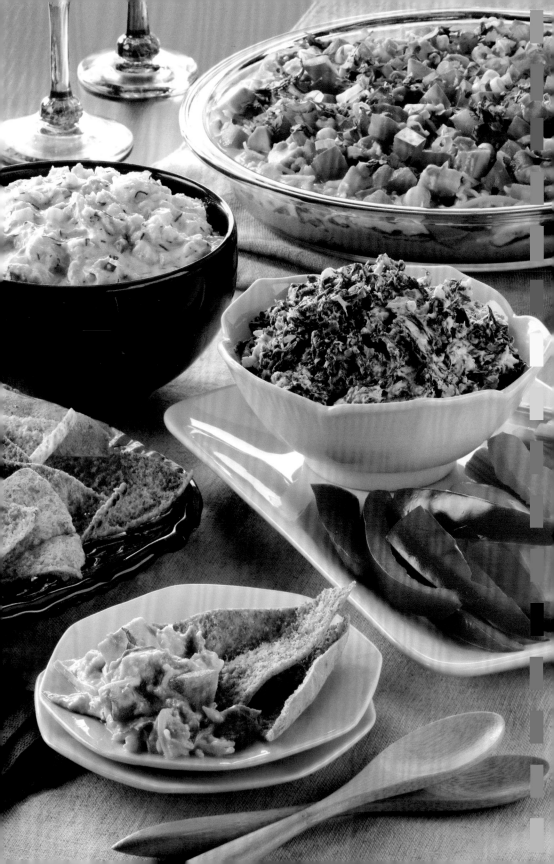

Spinach Dip

You can drastically reduce fat and calories by using yogurt cheese as the base of this popular dip. Make sure to buy yogurt without gelatin or modified starch because those yogurts won't drain well.

Low-fat plain yogurt (no gelatin)	2 cups	500 mL
Olive (or canola) oil	1 tsp.	5 mL
Finely chopped onion	1/2 cup	125 mL
Garlic clove, minced	1	1
(or 1/4 tsp., 1 mL, powder)		
Hot curry powder (optional)	1/2 tsp.	2 mL
Box of frozen spinach, thawed and	10 oz.	300 g
squeezed dry		
Salt	1/2 tsp.	2 mL
Pepper	1/4 tsp.	1 mL

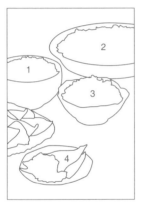

1. Seafood Garden Dip, page 20
2. Skinny Seven-Layer Dip, page 22
3. Spinach Dip, above
4. Crispy Baked Pita Chips, page 21

Props: Canhome Global

Line sieve with 3 coffee filters or double layer of cheesecloth. Set over large bowl. Pour yogurt into sieve. Let stand in refrigerator for 12 hours. Transfer yogurt cheese to medium bowl. Add 1/4 cup (60 mL) drained liquid. Stir. Discard remaining liquid.

Heat olive oil in medium frying pan on medium. Add onion. Cook for about 5 minutes, stirring often, until softened. Add garlic and curry powder. Heat and stir for about 1 minute until fragrant. Remove from heat.

Add remaining 3 ingredients. Stir. Let stand for about 15 minutes until cool. Add to yogurt cheese. Stir well. Chill, covered, for at least 1 hour. Makes about 1 3/4 cups (425 mL).

Pictured at left.

BEFORE: *1/4 cup (60 mL): **252 Calories**; 23.6 g Total Fat (11.9 Sat); 304 mg Sodium*

AFTER: *1/4 cup (60 mL): **38 Calories**; 1 g Total Fat (0 g Mono, 0 g Poly, 0 g Sat); 2 mg Cholesterol; 5 g Carbohydrate; 1 g Fibre; 2 g Protein; 248 mg Sodium*

Seafood Garden Dip

This delightfully tangy low-fat dip gets its creaminess from yogurt instead of cream cheese. Chock-full of fresh veggies that complement the shrimp and crabmeat.

Can of crabmeat, drained, cartilage removed, flaked	4 1/4 oz.	120 g
Cooked shrimp (peeled and deveined), chopped	4 oz.	113 g
Low-fat plain Balkan-style yogurt	2/3 cup	150 mL
Finely diced English cucumber (with peel)	1/3 cup	75 mL
Finely diced radish	1/4 cup	60 mL
Grated carrot	1/4 cup	60 mL
Mayonnaise	1/4 cup	60 mL
Chopped fresh dill (or 3/4 tsp., 4 mL, dried)	1 tbsp.	15 mL
Lemon juice	2 tsp.	10 mL
Chili paste (sambal oelek)	1/2 tsp.	2 mL
Grated lemon zest (see Tip, page 151)	1/2 tsp.	2 mL

Combine all 11 ingredients in medium bowl. Chill. Stir before serving. Makes about 2 1/3 cups (575 mL).

Pictured on page 18.

BEFORE: *1/4 cup (60 mL):* **274 Calories**; *25.2 g Total Fat (10.2 g Sat); 624 mg Sodium*

AFTER: *1/4 cup (60 mL):* **77 Calories**; *5 g Total Fat (0 g Mono, 0 g Poly, 1 g Sat); 35 mg Cholesterol; 2 g Carbohydrate; 0 g Fibre; 5 g Protein; 140 mg Sodium*

Chili Bean Nachos

These colourful nachos are topped with all the good stuff, and they're good for you, too! Serve with low-sodium salsa and low-fat sour cream if desired.

Diced orange pepper	1 1/2 cups	375 mL
Canned black beans, rinsed and drained	1 cup	250 mL
Sliced green onion	1/2 cup	125 mL
Chili powder	1 tbsp.	15 mL
Dried crushed chilies	1 tsp.	5 mL
Garlic powder	1/4 tsp.	1 mL
Bag of tortilla chips	11 1/4 oz.	320 g

(continued on next page)

Appetizers & Snacks

Grated jalapeño Monterey Jack cheese	1 1/2 cups	375 mL
Diced avocado	1/2 cup	125 mL
Diced seeded tomato	1/2 cup	125 mL

Combine first 6 ingredients in medium bowl.

Arrange half of chips on ungreased baking sheet with sides. Scatter half of orange pepper mixture over top.

Sprinkle with half of cheese. Repeat, layering with remaining chips, orange pepper mixture and cheese. Bake in 400°F (205°C) oven for about 10 minutes until cheese is melted.

Scatter avocado and tomato over top. Serves 8.

BEFORE: *1 serving: 486 Calories; 34 g Total Fat (**13 g Sat**); 656 mg Sodium*

AFTER: *1 serving: 310 Calories; 17 g Total Fat (1 g Mono, 0 g Poly, **4.5 g Sat**); 17 mg Cholesterol; 35 g Carbohydrate; 5 g Fibre; 9 g Protein; 428 mg Sodium*

Crispy Baked Pita Chips

An easy and quick alternative to potato chips. Excellent on their own or served with hummus or dip. Great for entertaining.

Garlic salt	1/2 tsp.	2 mL
Ground cumin	1/4 tsp.	1 mL
Onion powder	1/4 tsp.	1 mL
Pepper	1/4 tsp.	1 mL
Whole-wheat pita breads (7 inch, 18 cm, diameter) Cooking spray	4	4

Combine first 4 ingredients in small bowl.

Carefully split pita breads. Spray inside of rounds with cooking spray. Sprinkle with garlic salt mixture. Stack rounds. Cut into 8 wedges. Arrange in single layer on ungreased baking sheet with sides. Bake in 350°F (175°C) oven for about 8 minutes until crisp and golden. Makes 64 chips.

Pictured on page 18.

BEFORE: *16 chips: 280 Calories; **18 g Total Fat** (2 g Sat); 330 mg Sodium*

AFTER: *16 chips: 130 Calories; **1.5 g Total Fat** (0 g Mono, 0.5 g Poly, 0 g Sat); 0 mg Cholesterol; 28 g Carbohydrate; 4 g Fibre; 5 g Protein; 386 mg Sodium*

Skinny Seven-Layer Dip

Who doesn't love a good seven-layer dip? Serve this lower fat and sodium version with baked tortilla chips. If you choose a multi-grain or whole-wheat chip, that's even better!

Can of romano beans, rinsed and drained	19 oz.	540 mL
Canola oil	1 tbsp.	15 mL
Water	1 tbsp.	15 mL
Chili powder	2 tsp.	10 mL
Garlic clove, minced (or 1/4 tsp., 1 mL, powder)	1	1
Ground cumin	1/4 tsp.	1 mL
Chopped fresh spinach leaves, lightly packed	1 cup	250 mL
Non-fat plain yogurt	1 cup	250 mL
Hot salsa	1/4 cup	60 mL
Grated Mexican cheese blend	2/3 cup	150 mL
Diced avocado	1 cup	250 mL
Finely chopped pickled jalapeño peppers (see Tip, page 13)	1 tbsp.	15 mL
Lime juice	1 tbsp.	15 mL
Diced seeded Roma (plum) tomato	1 cup	250 mL
Thinly sliced green onion	2 tbsp.	30 mL
Chopped fresh cilantro (or parsley)	1 tbsp.	15 mL

BEFORE: *1 serving:*
253 Calories, 17 g Total Fat (11 g Sat); 3 g Fibre;
1232 mg Sodium

AFTER: *1 serving:*
166 Calories; 8 g Total Fat (3 g Mono, 1 g Poly, 2.5 g Sat);
10 mg Cholesterol;
17 g Carbohydrate;
7 g Fibre; 9 g Protein;
290 mg Sodium

Process first 6 ingredients in blender or food processor until almost smooth. Spread evenly in ungreased 9 inch (23 cm) pie plate.

Scatter spinach over bean mixture.

Stir yogurt and salsa in small bowl. Spread over spinach. Sprinkle with cheese.

Toss next 3 ingredients in small bowl. Scatter over cheese.

Layer remaining 3 ingredients, in order given, over avocado mixture. Serves 8.

Pictured on page 18.

Pear and Blue Cheese Slaw

Bacon, buttermilk and blue cheese combine for a boldly flavoured salad. Much lower in fat than the average coleslaw. Serve with slices of toasted sourdough.

Shredded cabbage, lightly packed	3 cups	750 mL
Julienned firm unpeeled pears (see Tip, below)	1 1/2 cups	375 mL
Julienned radish (see Tip, below)	1/2 cup	125 mL
Sliced green onion	2 tbsp.	30 mL
Bacon slices, cooked crisp and crumbled	4	4
1% buttermilk	1/3 cup	75 mL
Blue cheese, crumbled	1 oz.	28 g
Mayonnaise	1 tbsp.	15 mL
Dijon mustard	2 tsp.	10 mL
Coarsely ground pepper	1 tsp.	5 mL
Lemon juice	1 tsp.	5 mL

Toss first 5 ingredients in large bowl.

Whisk remaining 6 ingredients in small bowl. Add to cabbage mixture. Stir. Makes about 5 cups (1.25 L).

BEFORE: *1 cup (250 mL):* **489 Calories**; *47 g Total Fat (4.5 g Sat); 474 mg Sodium*

AFTER: *1 cup (250 mL):* **120 Calories**; *7 g Total Fat (1.5 g Mono, 0 g Poly, 2.5 g Sat); 15 mg Cholesterol; 11 g Carbohydrate; 3 g Fibre; 5 g Protein; 210 mg Sodium*

tip   To julienne, cut into very thin strips that resemble matchsticks.

Chicken Taco Salad

A great meal salad that's low in calories, fat and sodium. Serve with homemade or store-bought baked tortilla chips if desired.

Canola oil	1 tsp.	5 mL
Extra-lean ground chicken breast	3/4 lb.	340 g
Chili powder	2 tsp.	10 mL
Ground cumin	1/2 tsp.	2 mL
Garlic powder	1/4 tsp.	1 mL
Salsa	1/4 cup	60 mL
Cut or torn romaine lettuce, lightly packed	8 cups	2 L
Canned black beans, drained and rinsed	1 cup	250 mL
Slivered red pepper	1 cup	250 mL
Thinly sliced red onion	1/2 cup	125 mL
Light sour cream	1/4 cup	60 mL
Salsa	1/4 cup	60 mL
Lime juice	2 tbsp.	30 mL
Granulated sugar	1/2 tsp.	2 mL
Diced avocado	1 cup	250 mL
Diced tomato	1 cup	250 mL
Chopped fresh cilantro (or parsley)	2 tbsp.	30 mL

BEFORE: *1 cup (250 mL):* *479 Calories; 33.5 g Total Fat (4.5 g Sat);* **3051 mg Sodium**

AFTER: *1 cup (250 mL): 80 Calories; 3 g Total Fat (1.5 g Mono, 0 g Poly, 0.5 g Sat); 20 mg Cholesterol; 8 g Carbohydrate; 3 g Fibre; 8 g Protein;* **139 mg Sodium**

Heat canola oil in large frying pan on medium. Add next 4 ingredients. Scramble-fry for about 8 minutes until chicken is no longer pink. Add first amount of salsa. Stir. Remove from heat. Let stand for 10 minutes.

Toss next 4 ingredients in large bowl.

Stir next 4 ingredients in small bowl until smooth. Add to lettuce mixture. Toss.

Add remaining 3 ingredients and chicken mixture. Toss. Makes about 13 cups (3.25 L).

Salads & Soups

Vegetable Macaroni Salad

Classic summer fare. A pretty mix of colourful veggies and whole-wheat pasta,
lightly coated in a delightfully creamy vinaigrette.

Water	10 cups	2.5 L
Salt	1 tsp.	5 mL
Whole-wheat elbow macaroni	2 cups	500 mL
Diced seeded tomato	1 cup	250 mL
Sliced quartered small zucchini (with peel)	1 cup	250 mL
Diced red pepper	1/2 cup	125 mL
Frozen peas, thawed	1/2 cup	125 mL
Grated carrot	1/2 cup	125 mL
Sliced small fresh white mushrooms	1/2 cup	125 mL
Thinly sliced celery	1/2 cup	125 mL
CREAMY VINAIGRETTE		
Red wine vinegar	3 tbsp.	50 mL
Mayonnaise	2 tbsp.	30 mL
Canola oil	1 tbsp.	15 mL
Garlic clove, minced (or 1/4 tsp., 1 mL, powder)	1	1
Granulated sugar	1 tsp.	5 mL
Dried basil	1/2 tsp.	2 mL
Dried oregano	1/4 tsp.	1 mL
Dried thyme	1/4 tsp.	1 mL
Salt	1/4 tsp.	1 mL

BEFORE: *1 cup (250 mL): 302 Calories; 15.9 g Total Fat (1.2 g Sat);* **1 g Fibre***; 648 mg Sodium*

AFTER: *1 cup (250 mL): 160 Calories; 5 g Total Fat (1 g Mono, 0.5 g Poly, 0.5 g Sat); 1 mg Cholesterol; 26 g Carbohydrate;* **4 g Fibre***; 5 g Protein; 119 mg Sodium*

Combine water and salt in large saucepan. Bring to a boil. Add pasta. Boil, uncovered, for 8 to 10 minutes, stirring occasionally, until tender but firm. Drain. Rinse with cold water. Drain well. Transfer to large bowl.

Add next 7 ingredients.

Creamy Vinaigrette: Stir all 9 ingredients in small bowl. Makes about 1/3 cup (75 mL). Drizzle over vegetable mixture. Stir. Makes about 8 cups (2 L).

Roasted Garlic Caesar Salad

Roasted garlic adds a big punch of flavour to the dressing, so you don't have to add a ton of oil and sodium—which cuts way back on calories. You can make the croutons and dressing ahead of time and assemble the salad immediately before serving.

MULTI-GRAIN CROUTONS

Multi-grain (or whole-wheat) baguette, halved lengthwise	1/3	1/3
Garlic clove, halved	1	1

ROASTED GARLIC DRESSING

Garlic bulb	1	1
Olive oil	1 tsp.	5 mL
1% buttermilk	1/3 cup	75 mL
Lemon juice	2 tbsp.	30 mL
Dijon mustard	1 tsp.	5 mL
Granulated sugar	3/4 tsp.	4 mL
Grated lemon zest (see Tip, page 151)	1/2 tsp.	2 mL
Salt	1/4 tsp.	1 mL
Pepper	1/4 tsp.	1 mL

SALAD

Cut or torn romaine lettuce, lightly packed	8 cups	2 L
Grated Parmesan cheese	2 tbsp.	30 mL

BEFORE: *1 cup (250 mL):*
267 Calories;
24.2 g Total Fat (3.6 g Sat);
433 mg Sodium

AFTER: *1 cup (250 mL):*
64 Calories; *2 g Total Fat*
(0.5 g Mono, 0 g Poly,
0 g Sat); 2 mg Cholesterol;
10 g Carbohydrate;
3 g Fibre; 3 g Protein;
156 mg Sodium

Multi-Grain Croutons: Rub all sides of baguette with garlic. Cut into 3/4 inch (2 cm) cubes. Arrange in single layer on ungreased baking sheet with sides. Bake in 375°F (190°C) oven for about 12 minutes, stirring once, until golden and crisp. Let stand until cool. Makes about 2 cups (500 mL).

Roasted Garlic Dressing: Trim 1/4 inch (6 mm) from garlic bulb to expose tops of cloves, leaving bulb intact. Drizzle cut end with olive oil. Wrap loosely in greased foil. Bake in 375°F (190°C) oven for about 45 minutes until tender. Let stand until cool enough to handle. Squeeze garlic bulb to remove cloves from skin. Discard skin. Transfer garlic cloves to blender.

(continued on next page)

Add next 7 ingredients. Process until smooth. Makes about 1/2 cup (125 mL).

Salad: Toss lettuce and croutons in large bowl. Drizzle with dressing. Toss. Sprinkle with cheese. Makes about 9 cups (2.25 L).

Pictured on page 36.

Cheddar Broccoli Soup

This remake of the traditional favourite gets its creaminess from potatoes. Satisfying and very easy to prepare. Use gluten-free vegetable broth to make this soup gluten-free.

Canola oil	2 tsp.	10 mL
Chopped broccoli	4 cups	1 L
Chopped unpeeled potato	4 cups	1 L
Chopped onion	1 cup	250 mL
Garlic cloves, minced (or 1/2 tsp., 2 mL, powder)	2	2
Prepared vegetable broth	6 cups	1.5 L
Grated sharp Cheddar cheese	2/3 cup	150 mL
Grated Parmesan cheese	1/4 cup	60 mL
Dijon mustard	2 tsp.	10 mL
Pepper	1/4 tsp.	1 mL

BEFORE: *1 cup (250 mL):* **423 Calories**; *30.9 g Total Fat (16.8 g Sat); 1566 mg Sodium*

AFTER: *1 cup (250 mL):* **117 Calories**; *3.5 g Total Fat (1.5 g Mono, 0 g Poly, 1.5 g Sat); 8 mg Cholesterol; 17 g Carbohydrate; 2 g Fibre; 4 g Protein; 436 mg Sodium*

Heat canola oil in Dutch oven on medium. Add next 4 ingredients. Cook for about 10 minutes, stirring occasionally, until potato starts to soften.

Add broth. Bring to a boil. Reduce heat to medium-low. Simmer, covered, for about 20 minutes until potato is tender. Remove from heat. Carefully process with hand blender or in blender until smooth (see Safety Tip).

Add remaining 4 ingredients. Stir until cheese is melted. Makes about 9 1/2 cups (2.4 L).

Safety Tip: Follow manufacturer's instructions for processing hot liquids.

Summer Rice Salad

A chic rainbow of veggies adds a summery touch to the nutty flavour of wild rice. Wild rice is high in protein, low in fat and suitable for a gluten-free diet. Wild rice can also be cooked and then frozen.

Water	6 cups	1.5 L
Salt	1/8 tsp.	0.5 mL
Wild rice	3/4 cup	175 mL
Can of chickpeas (garbanzo beans), rinsed and drained	19 oz.	540 mL
Halved grape tomatoes	1 1/2 cups	375 mL
Chopped English cucumber (with peel), 1/2 inch (12 mm) pieces	1 cup	250 mL
Chopped yellow pepper	1 cup	250 mL
Chopped fresh basil	1/4 cup	60 mL
Sliced green onion	1/4 cup	60 mL
RED WINE VINAIGRETTE		
Red wine vinegar	1/4 cup	60 mL
Granulated sugar	1 tbsp.	15 mL
Dried oregano	1 tsp.	5 mL
Salt	1/2 tsp.	2 mL
Pepper	1/4 tsp.	1 mL
Olive oil	3 tbsp.	50 mL

BEFORE: *1 cup (250 mL):*
270 Calories; 12 g Total Fat (3 g Sat); **1 g Fibre***; 824 g Sodium*

AFTER: *1 cup (250 mL):*
167 Calories; 7 g Total Fat (4.5 g Mono, 1 g Poly, 1 g Sat); 0 mg Cholesterol; 26 g Carbohydrate; **4 g Fibre***; 6 g Protein; 256 mg Sodium*

Combine water and salt in small saucepan. Bring to a boil. Add rice. Reduce heat to medium. Boil, partially covered, for about 30 minutes until rice is tender. Drain well. Transfer to large bowl. Let stand for about 20 minutes, stirring occasionally, until cool.

Add next 6 ingredients. Stir.

Red Wine Vinaigrette: Stir first 5 ingredients in small bowl until sugar is dissolved. Add olive oil. Stir. Makes about 1/2 cup (125 mL). Drizzle over rice mixture. Toss. Makes about 7 cups (1.75 mL).

Pictured on page 36.

Salads & Soups

Lemon Ginger Noodle Salad

The bright, lemony dressing is definitely a winner. Cutting back on the amount of soy sauce used helps to reduce fat, and the whole-wheat pasta and veggies double the amount of fibre.

Water	10 cups	2.5 L
Salt	1 tsp.	5 mL
Whole-wheat spaghettini, broken in half	8 oz.	225 g
Broccoli slaw (or shredded cabbage with carrot)	1 1/2 cups	375 mL
Sliced trimmed snow peas, cut diagonally	1 cup	250 mL
Slivered red pepper	1/2 cup	125 mL
Slivered yellow pepper	1/2 cup	125 mL
Thinly sliced green onion	1/4 cup	60 mL
LEMON GINGER DRESSING		
Prepared chicken broth	1/4 cup	60 mL
Lemon juice	3 tbsp.	50 mL
Canola oil	1 tbsp.	15 mL
Finely grated ginger root (or 3/4 tsp., 4 mL, ground ginger)	1 tbsp.	15 mL
Liquid honey	1 tbsp.	15 mL
Soy sauce	1 tbsp.	15 mL
Grated lemon zest (see Tip, page 151)	1/2 tsp.	2 mL

BEFORE: *1 cup (250 mL): 238 Calories;* **10 g Total Fat** *(1 g Sat); 2 g Fibre; 376 mg Sodium*

AFTER: *1 cup (250 mL): 147 Calories;* **2 g Total Fat** *(1 g Mono, 0.5 g Poly, 0 g Sat); 0 mg Cholesterol; 28 g Carbohydrate; 4 g Fibre; 6 g Protein; 150 mg Sodium*

Combine water and salt in large saucepan. Bring to a boil. Add pasta. Boil, uncovered, for 5 to 8 minutes, stirring occasionally, until tender but firm. Drain. Rinse with cold water. Drain well. Transfer to large bowl.

Add next 5 ingredients. Toss.

Lemon Ginger Dressing: Whisk all 7 ingredients in small bowl. Makes about 3/4 cup (175 mL). Drizzle over noodle mixture. Toss. Makes about 7 1/2 cups (1.9 L) salad.

Pictured on page 36.

Wild Gumbo Soup

Wild rice has a lovely earthy flavour that sets this thick low-fat soup apart from the traditional gumbo—and also helps to reduce overall calories by nearly half.

Canola oil	1 tbsp.	15 mL
Chopped celery	1 1/2 cups	375 mL
Chopped green pepper	1 1/2 cups	375 mL
Chopped onion	1 1/2 cups	375 mL
Garlic cloves, minced (or 1/2 tsp., 2 mL, powder)	2	2
Dried oregano	1 tsp.	5 mL
Dried thyme	1 tsp.	5 mL
Dry mustard	1/2 tsp.	2 mL
Pepper	1/4 tsp.	1 mL
Prepared vegetable broth	6 cups	1.5 L
Sliced fresh (or frozen, thawed) okra, 1/2 inch (12 mm) thick	2 cups	500 mL
Diced kielbasa (or other spiced cooked lean sausage)	3/4 cup	175 mL
Wild rice	2/3 cup	150 mL
Bay leaves	2	2
Chopped cooked chicken breast	2 cups	500 mL
Chopped seeded tomato	1 cup	250 mL
Hot pepper sauce	1 tbsp.	15 mL

BEFORE: *1 cup (250 mL): 281 Calories;* **13.6 g Total Fat** *(1.1 g Sat); 677 g Sodium*

AFTER: *1 cup (250 mL): 150 Calories;* **4 g Total Fat** *(2.0 g Mono, 1.0 g Poly, 1.0 g Sat); 35 mg Cholesterol; 15 g Carbohydrate; 3 g Fibre; 14 g Protein; 458 mg Sodium*

Heat canola oil in Dutch oven on medium-high. Add next 8 ingredients. Cook for about 8 minutes, stirring occasionally, until onion is softened.

Add next 5 ingredients. Bring to a boil. Reduce heat to medium-low. Simmer, covered, for about 40 minutes until rice is tender. Remove and discard bay leaves.

Add remaining 3 ingredients. Stir. Cook, covered, for about 5 minutes until heated through. Makes about 10 cups (2.5 L).

Pictured on page 35.

Roasted Tomato Soup

(Gluten-free)

Navy beans bring a creamy texture to this charming tomato soup—without the fat of cream! Make this recipe gluten-free by using gluten-free vegetable broth.

Roma (plum) tomatoes, halved lengthwise	2 1/2 lbs.	1.1 kg
Coarsely chopped onion	2 cups	500 mL
Olive oil	1 tbsp.	15 mL
Garlic cloves, halved	2	2
Salt	1/4 tsp.	1 mL
Pepper	1/4 tsp.	1 mL
Prepared vegetable broth	6 cups	1.5 L
Can of navy beans, rinsed and drained	19 oz.	540 mL
Granulated sugar	1 tsp.	5 mL
Italian seasoning	1 tsp.	5 mL
Lemon juice	1 tsp.	5 mL

BEFORE: *1 cup (250 mL):*
138 Calories; 10 g Total Fat
(5 g Sat); 2 g Fibre;
508 mg Sodium

AFTER: *1 cup (250 mL):*
100 Calories; 2 g Total Fat
(1 g Mono, 0 g Poly,
0 g Sat); 0 mg Cholesterol;
18 g Carbohydrate;
4 g Fibre; 4 g Protein;
460 mg Sodium

Toss first 4 ingredients in large bowl. Arrange in single layer on greased baking sheet with sides. Sprinkle with salt and pepper. Bake in 350°F (175°C) oven for about 1 hour until tomato is soft and browned.

Combine next 4 ingredients in large saucepan or Dutch oven. Bring to a boil. Reduce heat to medium-low. Simmer, covered, for 15 minutes. Remove from heat.

Add lemon juice and tomato mixture. Stir. Carefully process in blender or food processor in batches until smooth (see Safety Tip). Makes about 10 1/2 cups (2.6 L).

Pictured on page 35.

Safety Tip: Follow manufacturer's instructions for processing hot liquids.

Paré Pointer

Mist is what we get when the rain doesn't feel like trying.

Hamburger Soup

You'll be enjoying hearty soup before you know it when you pull out these ingredients. The quick cooking time is remarkable for such a full-flavoured soup.

Canola oil	1 tsp.	5 mL
Extra-lean ground beef	3/4 lb.	340 g
Chopped onion	1 cup	250 mL
Diced celery	1 cup	250 mL
Low-sodium prepared beef broth	8 cups	2 L
Frozen mixed vegetables	3 cups	750 mL
Can of diced tomatoes (with juice)	28 oz.	796 mL
Can of black beans, rinsed and drained	19 oz.	540 mL
Tomato paste (see Tip, below)	3 tbsp.	50 mL
Italian seasoning	1 tsp.	5 mL
Dried crushed chilies	1/4 tsp.	1 mL
Whole-wheat elbow macaroni	1/2 cup	125 mL

BEFORE: *1 cup (250 mL): 207 Calories;* **12 g Total Fat** *(5 g Sat); 780 mg Sodium*

AFTER: *1 cup (250 mL): 100 Calories;* **1 g Total Fat** *(0.5 g Mono, 0 g Poly, 0.5 g Sat); 14 mg Cholesterol; 14 g Carbohydrate; 3 g Fibre; 9 g Protein; 555 mg Sodium*

Heat canola oil in Dutch oven on medium. Add next 3 ingredients. Scramble-fry for about 10 minutes until beef starts to brown.

Add next 7 ingredients. Bring to a boil.

Add pasta. Stir. Simmer, covered, for about 8 minutes, stirring occasionally, until pasta is tender but firm. Makes about 15 1/3 cups (3.8 L).

Pictured on page 35.

 tip If a recipe calls for less than an entire can of tomato paste, freeze the unopened can for 30 minutes. Open both ends and push the contents through one end. Slice off only what you need. Freeze the remaining paste in a resealable freezer bag or plastic wrap for future use.

Three-Mushroom Beef Stroganoff

Lots of rich-tasting, mushroom-flavoured sauce that could also be served along with rice, noodles or potatoes.

Prepared beef broth	2 cups	500 mL
Package of dried porcini mushrooms	1/2 oz.	14 g
Butter	2 tsp.	10 mL
Beef top sirloin steak, trimmed of fat and thinly sliced	3/4 lb.	340 g
Sliced onion	1 cup	250 mL
Garlic clove, minced (or 1/4 tsp., 1 mL, powder)	1	1
Pepper	1/4 tsp.	1 mL
Sliced fresh brown (or white) mushrooms	2 cups	500 mL
Sliced portobello mushrooms, gills removed (see Note)	2 cups	500 mL
All-purpose flour	2 tbsp.	30 mL
Sour cream	2 tbsp.	30 mL

BEFORE: *3/4 cup (175 mL):* **368 Calories**; *26.7 g Total Fat (10.4 Sat); 742 mg Sodium*

AFTER: *3/4 cup (175 mL):* **180 Calories**; *7 g Total Fat (2.5 g Mono, 0 g Poly, 3 g Sat); 39 mg Cholesterol; 10 g Carbohydrate; 2 g Fibre; 20 g Protein; 335 mg Sodium*

Bring broth to a boil in small saucepan. Add porcini mushrooms. Remove from heat. Let stand, covered, for 10 minutes. Remove mushrooms. Strain mushroom liquid through double layer of cheesecloth into small bowl. Chop porcini mushrooms.

Melt butter in large frying pan on medium. Add next 4 ingredients. Cook for about 8 minutes, stirring occasionally, until beef is no longer pink.

Add brown, portobello and porcini mushrooms. Cook for about 15 minutes, stirring occasionally, until mushrooms are browned and liquid is evaporated.

Sprinkle with flour. Heat and stir for 1 minute. Slowly add mushroom liquid, stirring constantly until boiling and thickened. Remove from heat.

Stir in sour cream. Makes about 3 1/2 cups (875 mL).

Note: Because the gills can sometimes be bitter, make sure to remove them from the portobellos. Scrape out and discard the gills with a small spoon.

Salsa Beef Tacos

Adding black beans, coleslaw and salsa to the ground beef bulks up the portion size while still keeping everything lean. These flavourful offerings are much lower in saturated fat than standard tacos.

Canola oil	1 tsp.	5 mL
Extra-lean ground beef	1/2 lb.	225 g
Finely chopped onion	1 cup	250 mL
Chili powder	2 tsp.	10 mL
Canned black beans, rinsed and drained, coarsely mashed	1 cup	250 mL
Coleslaw mix	1 cup	250 mL
Hot salsa	1/2 cup	125 mL
Hard taco shells	8	8
Diced tomato	1/2 cup	125 mL
Grated Mexican cheese blend	1/2 cup	125 mL

Heat canola oil in large frying pan on medium. Add next 3 ingredients. Scramble-fry for about 10 minutes until beef is browned.

Add next 3 ingredients. Cook for about 2 minutes, stirring occasionally, until heated through. Transfer to medium bowl.

Arrange taco shells on ungreased baking sheet. Bake in 400°F (205°C) oven for about 5 minutes until warm. Spoon beef mixture into shells.

Sprinkle with tomato and cheese. Makes 8 tacos.

Pictured on page 72 and on back cover.

BEFORE: *1 taco:* **320 Calories**; *22 g Total Fat (10 g Sat); 589 mg Sodium*

AFTER: *1 taco:* **150 Calories**; *7 g Total Fat (1.5 g Mono, 0 g Poly, 2.5 g Sat); 21 mg Cholesterol; 14 g Carbohydrate; 3 g Fibre; 9 g Protein; 285 mg Sodium*

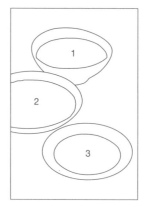

1. Wild Gumbo Soup, page 30
2. Roasted Tomato Soup, page 31
3. Hamburger Soup, page 32

Props: Casa Bugatti

Beef

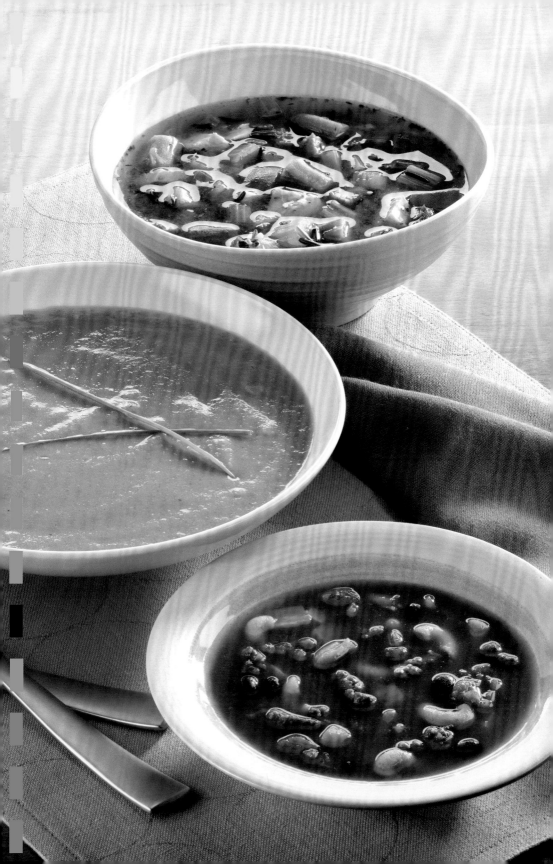

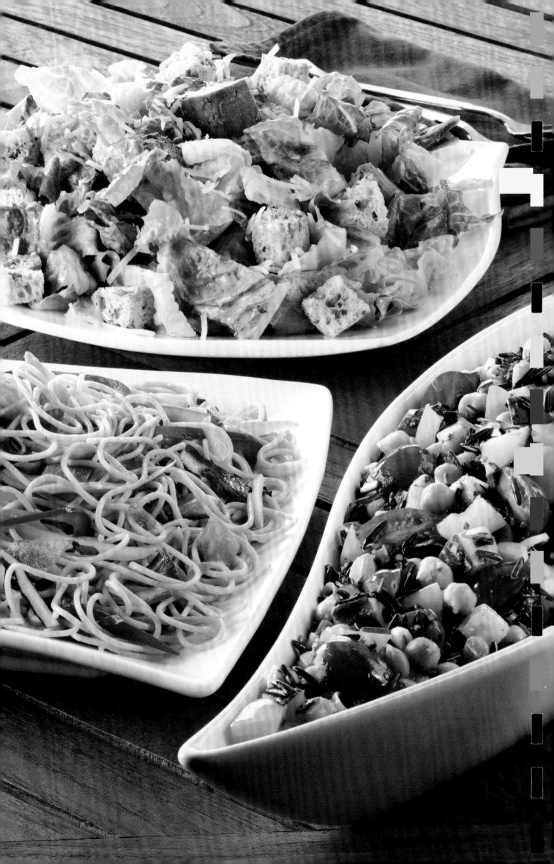

Sweet and Sour Meatballs

Preparing your own sweet-and-sour sauce results in lower fat and fewer calories than using store-bought sauce. You can make this recipe gluten-free by using gluten-free soy sauce.

Cooked long-grain brown rice (about 1/4 cup, 60 mL, uncooked)	1 cup	250 mL
Finely chopped canned water chestnuts	1/4 cup	60 mL
Grated onion	1/4 cup	60 mL
Salt	1/4 tsp.	1 mL
Pepper	1/2 tsp.	2 mL
Lean ground beef	3/4 lb.	340 g
Can of crushed pineapple (with juice)	14 oz.	398 mL
Apricot jam	1/4 cup	60 mL
Rice vinegar	2 tbsp.	30 mL
Soy sauce	2 tbsp.	30 mL
Cornstarch	1 tbsp.	15 mL
Finely grated ginger root (or 1/2 tsp., 2 mL, ground ginger)	2 tsp	10 mL

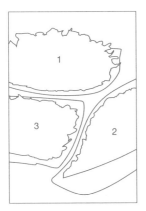

1. Roasted Garlic Caesar Salad, page 26
2. Summer Rice Salad, page 28
3. Lemon Ginger Noodle Salad, page 29

Props: Moderno
Danesco

Combine first 5 ingredients in large bowl. Add beef. Mix well. Shape into 1 inch (2.5 cm) balls. Arrange in single layer on greased baking sheet with sides. Cook in 400°F (205°C) oven for about 15 minutes until no longer pink inside. Makes about 31 meatballs.

Combine remaining 6 ingredients in large saucepan. Bring to a boil. Reduce heat to medium-low. Boil gently, uncovered, for about 5 minutes, stirring often, until thickened. Add meatballs. Stir gently until coated. Makes about 4 cups (1 L).

Pictured on page 53.

BEFORE: *1/2 cup (125 mL): 333 Calories;* **22 g Total Fat** *(8 g Sat); 388 mg Sodium*

AFTER: *1/2 cup (125 mL): 187 Calories;* **6 g Total Fat** *(2.5 g Mono, 0 g Poly, 2 g Sat); 25 mg Cholesterol; 20 g Carbohydrate; 1 g Fibre; 10 g Protein; 340 mg Sodium*

Beef

Skinny Shepherd's Pie

Steak sauce adds a distinctive flavour to this low-fat shepherd's pie.
Serve with a leafy green salad.

Chopped peeled potato	4 cups	1 L
Light sour cream	1/2 cup	125 mL
Chopped fresh chives (or 3/4 tsp., 4 mL, dried)	1 tbsp.	15 mL
Salt	1/4 tsp.	1 mL
Canola oil	2 tsp.	10 mL
Extra-lean ground beef	3/4 lb.	340 g
Chopped onion	1 cup	250 mL
Finely chopped carrot	1 cup	250 mL
Prepared beef broth	1 1/2 cups	375 mL
Steak sauce	2 tbsp.	30 mL
Pepper	1/4 tsp.	1 mL
Bulgur, fine grind	1/2 cup	125 mL
Frozen peas, thawed	1 cup	250 mL

BEFORE: *1 serving:*
*369 Calories; **17.6 g Total Fat** (5.3 g Sat);*
918 mg Sodium

AFTER: *1 serving:*
*280 Calories; **6 g Total Fat** (2 g Mono, 0.5 g Poly, 2 g Sat);*
38 mg Cholesterol;
41 g Carbohydrate;
5 g Fibre; 19 g Protein;
454 mg Sodium

Pour water into large saucepan until about 1 inch (2.5 cm) deep. Add potato. Cover. Bring to a boil. Reduce heat to medium. Boil gently, covered, for 12 to 15 minutes until tender. Drain. Add next 3 ingredients. Mash. Cover to keep warm.

Heat canola oil in large frying pan on medium. Add next 3 ingredients. Scramble-fry for 10 minutes until beef is browned.

Add next 3 ingredients. Bring to a boil. Add bulgur. Stir. Cook, covered, for about 10 minutes until bulgur is tender and liquid is almost absorbed.

Add peas. Stir. Transfer to ungreased shallow 2 quart (2 L) baking dish. Spread mashed potatoes over beef mixture. Bake, uncovered, in 350°F (175°C) oven for about 30 minutes until heated through and bubbling at edges. Serves 6.

Mexi Meatloaf

This tender low-fat meatloaf is topped with salsa and Mexican cheese.
If desired, use an egg instead of the flaxseed and water.

Ground flaxseed (see Tip, below)	2 tbsp.	30 mL
Warm water	1/4 cup	60 mL
Can of black beans, rinsed and drained	19 oz.	540 mL
Frozen kernel corn, thawed and chopped	1 cup	250 mL
Finely chopped onion	1/2 cup	125 mL
Yellow cornmeal	1/2 cup	125 mL
Chili powder	2 tbsp.	30 mL
Granulated sugar	1 tsp.	5 mL
Garlic cloves, minced (or 1/2 tsp., 2 mL, powder)	2	2
Salt	1/4 tsp.	1 mL
Extra-lean ground beef	3/4 lb.	340 g
Salsa	1/2 cup	125 mL
Grated Mexican cheese blend	1/2 cup	125 mL

BEFORE: *1 wedge:*
312 Calories; **19.4 g Total**
Fat *(8.8 g Sat); 1.5 g Fibre;*
716 Sodium

AFTER: *1 wedge:*
189 Calories; **5 g Total**
Fat *(1 g Mono, 0.5 g Poly,*
2.5 g Sat);
33 mg Cholesterol;
22 g Carbohydrate;
4 g Fibre; 14 g Protein;
384 mg Sodium

Combine flaxseed and water in large bowl. Let stand for 5 minutes.

Mash 1 cup (250 mL) beans in small bowl. Add to flaxseed mixture. Add next 7 ingredients and remaining beans. Stir.

Add beef. Mix well. Press evenly into greased 9 inch (23 cm) pie plate. Bake in 350°F (175°C) oven for about 45 minutes until internal temperature reaches 160°F (71°C).

Spread salsa over meatloaf. Sprinkle with cheese. Bake for about 10 minutes until cheese is melted. Cuts into 8 wedges.

 Whole flaxseed may be ground in a blender or coffee grinder. Store in airtight container in the refrigerator.

Ground flaxseed is digested more readily than whole flaxseed, which simply passes through the body. Grinding the seeds just before using them best preserves flavour and nutrition, but pre-ground seeds are more convenient.

Beef Lentil Lasagna

Adding lentils to lasagna is a great way to reduce fat and increase fibre while still keeping a healthy and satisfying portion size.

Canola oil	2 tsp.	10 mL
Chopped fresh brown (or white) mushrooms	2 cups	500 mL
Extra-lean ground beef	1/2 lb.	225 g
Chopped onion	1 cup	250 mL
Garlic cloves, minced (or 1/2 tsp., 2 mL, powder)	2	2
Can of diced tomatoes (with juice)	28 oz.	796 mL
Can of lentils, rinsed and drained	19 oz.	540 mL
Can of crushed tomatoes	14 oz.	398 mL
Water	1 cup	250 mL
Italian seasoning	1 tbsp.	15 mL
Granulated sugar	1 tsp.	5 mL
Pepper	1/2 tsp.	2 mL
Dried crushed chilies (optional)	1/2 tsp.	2 mL
Large egg	1	1
Light ricotta cheese	2 cups	500 mL
Box of frozen chopped spinach, thawed and squeezed dry	10 oz.	300 g
Grated Parmesan cheese	1/2 cup	125 mL
Oven-ready whole-grain lasagna noodles	9	9
Grated part-skim mozzarella cheese	2 cups	500 mL

BEFORE: *1 piece:*
*503 Calories; 26.9 g Total Fat (13.3 Sat); **1 g Fibre**; 695 mg Sodium*

AFTER: *1 piece:*
*290 Calories; 11 g Total Fat (3.5 g Mono, 0.5 g Poly, 6 g Sat); 48 mg Cholesterol; 29 g Carbohydrate; **5 g Fibre**; 22 g Protein; 660 mg Sodium*

Heat canola oil in large frying pan on medium. Add next 4 ingredients. Scramble-fry for about 12 minutes until onion is softened and liquid from mushrooms is evaporated.

Add next 8 ingredients. Bring to a boil. Reduce heat to medium-low. Cook, partially covered, for 15 minutes.

Combine next 4 ingredients in medium bowl.

(continued on next page)

Beef

To assemble, layer ingredients in greased 9 x 13 inch (23 x 33 cm) baking dish as follows:

1. 1 cup (250 mL) tomato mixture
2. 3 noodles
3. Half of ricotta cheese mixture
4. Half of remaining tomato mixture
5. 3 noodles
6. Remaining ricotta cheese mixture
7. Remaining noodles
8. Remaining tomato mixture

Bake, covered, in 350°F (175°C) oven for about 45 minutes until noodles are tender. Remove foil. Sprinkle with mozzarella cheese. Bake, uncovered, for about 20 minutes until cheese is golden. Let stand for 10 minutes. Cuts into 12 pieces.

Paré Pointer

Convicts talk so slow. It can take twenty-five years to finish a sentence.

Beef

Chipotle Squash Chili

A hearty and colourful chili dish that's sure to please. Chipotle peppers add a hint of smoky heat, and squash provides some complementary sweetness.

Canola oil	1 tbsp.	15 mL
Extra-lean ground beef	3/4 lb.	340 g
Chopped celery	1 cup	250 mL
Chopped onion	1 cup	250 mL
Diced carrot	1 cup	250 mL
Garlic cloves, minced (or 1/2 tsp., 2 mL, powder)	2	2
Can of diced tomatoes (with juice)	28 oz.	796 mL
Chopped butternut squash	3 cups	750 mL
Can of black beans, rinsed and drained	19 oz.	540 mL
Can of red kidney beans, rinsed and drained	14 oz.	398 mL
Tomato paste (see Tip, page 32)	1/4 cup	60 mL
Chili powder	2 tbsp.	30 mL
Finely chopped chipotle peppers in adobo sauce (see Tip, page 128)	2 tsp.	10 mL
Pepper	1/4 tsp.	1 mL
Diced red pepper	1 cup	250 mL
Frozen kernel corn, thawed	1 cup	250 mL

BEFORE: *1 cup (250 mL):*
299 Calories; 8.9 g Total Fat (5 g Sat);
1252 mg Sodium

AFTER: *1 cup (250 mL):*
186 Calories; 4.5 g Total Fat (1.5 g Mono, 0.5 g Poly, 1 g Sat); 20 mg Cholesterol; 28 g Carbohydrate; 7 g Fibre; 13 g Protein;
464 mg Sodium

Heat canola oil in Dutch oven on medium-high. Add beef. Scramble-fry for about 5 minutes until no longer pink. Reduce heat to medium.

Add next 4 ingredients. Cook for about 12 minutes, stirring occasionally, until celery is softened.

Add next 8 ingredients. Stir. Bring to a boil. Reduce heat to medium-low. Simmer, covered, for about 40 minutes, stirring occasionally, until squash is tender.

Add red pepper and corn. Stir. Cook, covered, for about 5 minutes, stirring occasionally, until red pepper is tender-crisp. Makes about 10 cups (2.5 L).

Beef

Beef and Bean Casserole

A healthy, flavourful version of hamburger casserole. The medley of
Italian-themed vegetables adds fibre and reduces calories to less than half.

Water	8 cups	2 L
Salt	1 tsp.	5 mL
Whole-wheat elbow macaroni	1 1/2 cups	375 mL
Canola oil	1 tsp.	5 mL
Extra-lean ground beef	1/2 lb.	225 g
Chopped red onion	1 cup	250 mL
Garlic cloves, minced (or 1/2 tsp., 2 mL, powder)	2	2
Chopped tomato	2 cups	500 mL
Chopped fresh spinach leaves, lightly packed	1 1/2 cups	375 mL
Diced zucchini (with peel)	1 1/2 cups	375 mL
Can of mixed beans, rinsed and drained	19 oz.	540 mL
Can of tomato sauce	7 1/2 oz.	213 mL
Balsamic vinegar	1 tbsp.	15 mL
Italian seasoning	1 tsp.	5 mL
Pepper	1/4 tsp.	1 mL
Grated Parmesan cheese	1 cup	250 mL

BEFORE: *1 cup (250 mL):*
446 Calories; 17.3 g Total
Fat (8.8 g Sat); **1 g Fibre**;
829 mg Sodium

AFTER: *1 cup (250 mL):*
205 Calories; 4.5 g Total
Fat (1.5 g Mono,
0.5 g Poly, 2 g Sat);
23 mg Cholesterol;
29 g Carbohydrate;
6 g Fibre; *15 g Protein;*
374 mg Sodium

Combine water and salt in large saucepan. Bring to a boil. Add pasta. Boil, uncovered, for 6 minutes, stirring occasionally. Drain, reserving 1 cup (250 mL) cooking liquid.

Heat canola oil in large frying pan on medium-high. Add next 3 ingredients. Scramble-fry for about 5 minutes until beef is no longer pink and onion is softened.

Add next 8 ingredients. Stir. Cook for about 5 minutes until heated through. Add to pasta. Add reserved cooking liquid. Stir. Transfer to greased 9 x 13 inch (23 x 33 cm) baking dish.

Sprinkle with cheese. Bake in 375°F (190°C) oven for about 30 minutes until bubbling and heated through. Makes about 8 cups (2 L).

Prairie Burgers

With a homemade chutney, you get all the flavour without all the extra calories of prepared condiments.

SPICED RHUBARB CHUTNEY

Canola oil	1/2 tsp.	2 mL
Chopped fresh (or frozen, thawed) rhubarb	3/4 cups	175 mL
Diced peeled cooking apple (such as McIntosh)	2/3 cup	150 mL
Chopped onion	1/4 cup	60 mL
Apple cider vinegar	1 tbsp.	15 mL
Liquid honey	1 tbsp.	15 mL
Dried sage	1/4 tsp.	1 mL
Ground allspice	1/4 tsp.	1 mL

MUSHROOM SAGE BURGERS

Large egg	1	1
Quick-cooking rolled oats (not instant)	1/3 cup	75 mL
Chopped fresh white mushrooms	1/2 cup	125 mL
Grated carrot	1/4 cup	60 mL
Dried sage	1/4 tsp.	1 mL
Dried thyme	1/4 tsp.	1 mL
Salt	1/4 tsp.	1 mL
Pepper	1/4 tsp.	1 mL
Extra-lean ground beef	1 lb.	454 g
Whole-grain bread slices (about 1 inch, 2.5 cm, thick, each)	4	4

BEFORE: *1 serving:*
*771 Calories; 45 g Total Fat (**16 g Sat**); 970 mg Sodium*

AFTER: *1 serving:*
*380 Calories; 10 g Total Fat (3.5 g Mono, 1 g Poly, **3 g Sat**); 105 mg Cholesterol; 47 g Carbohydrate; 7 g Fibre; 34 g Protein; 540 mg Sodium*

Spiced Rhubarb Chutney: Heat canola oil in medium saucepan on medium. Add next 3 ingredients. Cook for about 8 minutes, stirring often, until rhubarb and apple are softened.

Add remaining 4 ingredients. Stir. Cook, uncovered, on medium-low for 5 minutes, stirring occasionally, to blend flavours. Remove from heat. Makes about 7/8 cup (200 mL) chutney.

(continued on next page)

Mushroom Sage Burgers: Combine first 8 ingredients in large bowl. Add ground beef. Mix well. Divide into 4 equal portions. Shape into 1/2 inch (12 mm) thick patties. Preheat gas barbecue to medium (see Tip, below). Place patties on greased grill. Close lid. Cook for about 7 minutes per side until internal temperature reaches 160°F (71°C). Remove to large plate. Cover to keep warm.

Toast bread slices on greased grill. Place 1 bread slice on each of 4 dinner plates. Place 1 patty on top of each bread slice. Serve with chutney on the side or spooned on top of patties. Serves 4.

 Too cold to barbecue? Use the broiler instead! Your food should cook in about the same length of time—and remember to turn or baste as directed. Set your oven rack so that the food is about 3 to 4 inches (7.5 to 10 cm) away from the top element—for most ovens, this is the top rack.

Beefy Mushroom Pizza

With pizza, keeping calories down is all about proportion and using healthier ingredients. Whole-wheat flour and flaxseed add fibre to the crust, and mushrooms help to "beef" up portions to leave you feeling satisfied.

All-purpose flour	3/4 cup	175 mL
Whole-wheat flour	3/4 cup	175 mL
Flaxseed	2 tbsp.	30 mL
Envelope of instant yeast (or 2 1/4 tsp., 11 mL)	1/4 oz.	8 g
Salt	1 tsp.	5 mL
Granulated sugar	1/2 tsp.	2 mL
Very warm water (see Tip, page 47)	2/3 cup	150 mL
Canola oil	1 tbsp.	15 mL
Canola oil	1 tsp.	5 mL
Extra-lean ground beef	1/2 lb.	225 g
Sliced fresh white mushrooms	1 1/2 cups	375 mL
Chopped onion	1/2 cup	125 mL
Steak sauce	2 tbsp.	30 mL
Dried crushed chilies	1/2 tsp.	2 mL
Tomato sauce	1/2 cup	125 mL
Diced red pepper	1/2 cup	125 mL
Grated sharp Cheddar cheese	1 cup	250 mL

BEFORE: *1 wedge:*
398 Calories; *23 g Total Fat (11 g Sat); 1 g Fibre; 1170 mg Sodium*

AFTER: *1 wedge:*
220 Calories; *9 g Total Fat (3.5 g Mono, 1.5 g Poly, 3.5 g Sat); 25 mg Cholesterol; 23 g Carbohydrate; 3 g Fibre; 13 g Protein; 520 mg Sodium*

Combine first 6 ingredients in extra-large bowl. Make a well in centre.

Add water and first amount of canola oil to well. Stir until soft dough forms. Turn out onto lightly floured surface. Knead for about 5 minutes until smooth and elastic. Place in greased large bowl, turning once to grease top. Cover with greased waxed paper and tea towel. Let stand at room temperature for 15 minutes. Turn out onto lightly floured surface. Roll out dough to 12 inch (30 cm) circle. Transfer to 12 inch (30 cm) greased pizza pan.

Heat second amount of canola oil in medium frying pan on medium. Add next 5 ingredients. Scramble-fry for about 12 minutes until beef is browned and liquid is evaporated.

(continued on next page)

Spread tomato sauce over dough. Scatter beef mixture over sauce. Sprinkle with red pepper and cheese. Bake on bottom rack in 450°F (230°C) oven for about 18 minutes until crust is golden and cheese is melted. Cuts into 8 wedges.

Pictured on page 107.

Lazy Cabbage Roll Bake

This recipe remake skips the canned soup and uses healthy brown rice, which increases fibre. A pleasing casserole with a comforting, tomato-tinted appearance.

Canola oil	2 tsp.	10 mL
Extra-lean ground beef	1 lb.	454 g
Chopped celery	1 cup	250 mL
Chopped onion	1 cup	250 mL
Can of diced tomatoes (with juice)	14 oz.	398 mL
Can of tomato sauce	14 oz.	398 mL
Long-grain brown rice	1 cup	250 mL
Water	1 cup	250 mL
Pepper	1/2 tsp.	2 mL
Shredded cabbage, lightly packed	5 cups	1.25 L
Grated carrot	1 cup	250 mL

BEFORE: *1 cup (250 mL):*
***442 Calories**; 25 g Total Fat (10 g Sat); 2 g Fibre; 613 mg Sodium*

AFTER: *1 cup (250 mL):*
***220 Calories**; 4.5 g Total Fat (2 g Mono, 0.5 g Poly, 1.5 g Sat); 35 mg Cholesterol; 30 g Carbohydrate; 5 g Fibre; 16 g Protein; 554 mg Sodium*

Heat canola oil in large frying pan on medium. Add next 3 ingredients. Scramble-fry for about 10 minutes until celery is softened.

Add next 5 ingredients. Heat and stir until boiling. Transfer to greased 9 x 13 inch (23 x 33 cm) baking dish.

Scatter cabbage and carrot over beef mixture. Bake, covered, in 350°F (175°C) oven for about 1 1/2 hours, stirring at halftime, until rice is tender. Let stand, covered, for 10 minutes. Makes about 8 cups (2 L).

tip When using yeast, it is important for the liquid to be at the correct temperature. If the liquid is too cool, the yeast will not activate properly. If the liquid is too hot, the yeast will be destroyed. For best results, follow the recommended temperatures as instructed on the package.

Beef

Barley Beef Stew

A comfort classic at its tender, melt-in-your-mouth best. The addition of fibre-rich barley and the abundance of vegetables make this a balanced, all-in-one dish.

Canola oil	1 tbsp.	15 mL
Stewing beef, trimmed of fat	1 1/2 lbs.	680 g
Salt, sprinkle		
Pepper, sprinkle		
Low-sodium prepared beef broth	3 cups	750 mL
Pot barley	1/2 cup	125 mL
Balsamic vinegar	1 tbsp.	15 mL
Garlic cloves, minced (or 1/2 tsp., 2 mL, powder)	2	2
Sprig of fresh rosemary (or 1 tsp., 5 mL, dried, crushed)	1	1
Baby carrots	2 cups	500 mL
Cubed butternut squash (1 inch, 2.5 cm, pieces)	2 cups	500 mL
Halved baby potatoes	2 cups	500 mL
Chopped onion	2 cups	500 mL

BEFORE: *1 cup (250 mL): 531 Calories;* ***25.9 g Total Fat*** *(7.8 g Sat); 5 g Fibre; 662 mg Sodium*

AFTER: *1 cup (250 mL): 278 Calories;* ***8 g Total Fat*** *(3.5 g Mono, 1 g Poly, 2.5 g Sat); 40 mg Cholesterol; 29 g Carbohydrate; 4 g Fibre; 23 g Protein; 340 mg Sodium*

Heat canola oil in large frying pan on medium-high. Add beef. Sprinkle with salt and pepper. Cook for about 5 minutes, stirring occasionally, until browned. Transfer to greased 4 quart (4 L) casserole.

Add next 5 ingredients to same frying pan. Bring to a boil, stirring and scraping any brown bits from bottom of pan. Add to beef. Stir.

Layer remaining 4 ingredients in order given over beef mixture. Do not stir. Cook, covered, in 350°F (175°C) oven for about 2 3/4 hours until beef is tender. Makes about 8 cups (2 L).

Pictured on page 53.

Paré Pointer

Would a skinny parrot be Polly-unsaturated?

Beef Pot Pie

This amazing pot pie is lower in calories, fat and sodium! The phyllo pastry helps lighten things up and creates an attractive ruffled topping to boot.

Canola oil	1 tsp.	5 mL
Chopped celery	1 cup	250 mL
Chopped onion	1 cup	250 mL
Finely chopped carrot	1 cup	250 mL
All-purpose flour	1 tbsp.	15 mL
Prepared beef broth	1 cup	250 mL
Chopped cooked roast beef	2 cups	500 mL
Chopped Swiss chard, lightly packed	2 cups	500 mL
Tomato paste (see Tip, page 32)	1 tbsp.	15 mL
Dried oregano	1/2 tsp.	2 mL
Pepper	1/4 tsp.	1 mL
Phyllo pastry sheets, thawed according to package directions	4	4
Cooking spray		

BEFORE: *1 serving:*
*660 Calories; 37 g Total Fat (**11 g Sat**); 720 mg Sodium*

AFTER: *1 serving:*
*257 Calories; 6 g Total Fat (2.5 g Mono, 1 g Poly, **1.5 g Sat**); 40 mg Cholesterol; 24 g Carbohydrate; 3 g Fibre; 26 g Protein; 433 mg Sodium*

Heat canola oil in large frying pan on medium. Add next 3 ingredients. Cook for about 10 minutes, stirring often, until celery is softened.

Sprinkle with flour. Heat and stir for 1 minute. Slowly add broth, stirring constantly until boiling and thickened.

Add next 5 ingredients. Cook for about 5 minutes, stirring occasionally, until heated through. Transfer to greased 2 quart (2 L) casserole.

Place 1 pastry sheet on work surface. Cover remaining sheets with damp towel to prevent drying. Spray pastry sheet with cooking spray. Bunch up loosely. Place over beef mixture. Repeat with remaining pastry sheets and cooking spray. Bake in 375°F (190°C) oven for about 25 minutes until pastry is golden. Serves 4.

Pictured on page 53.

Macaroni Sausage Frittata

There's no need to give up pasta or Parmesan cheese when you use whole-wheat macaroni and lighter ingredients.

Water	4 cups	1 L
Salt	1/2 tsp.	2 mL
Whole-wheat elbow macaroni	1 cup	250 mL
Canola oil	1 tsp.	5 mL
Turkey (or chicken) sausages, cut into 1/2 inch (12 mm) pieces	4	4
Chopped onion	1/2 cup	125 mL
Cajun seasoning	1 tsp.	5 mL
Egg whites (large)	3	3
Large eggs	2	2
1% buttermilk	1/2 cup	125 mL
Grated Parmesan cheese	1/4 cup	60 mL

BEFORE: *1 wedge:*
*481 Calories; 32 g Total Fat (**16 g Sat**); 839 mg Sodium*

AFTER: *1 wedge:*
*246 Calories; 8 g Total Fat (3 g Mono, 1.5 g Poly, **2 g Sat**); 102 mg Cholesterol; 25 g Carbohydrate; 3 g Fibre; 18 g Protein; 630 mg Sodium*

Combine water and salt in large saucepan. Bring to a boil. Add pasta. Boil, uncovered, for 8 to 10 minutes, stirring occasionally, until tender but firm. Drain. Return to same pot. Cover to keep warm.

Heat canola oil in large frying pan on medium. Add next 3 ingredients. Cook for about 5 minutes, stirring often, until sausage is browned. Drain. Add pasta. Stir. Spread evenly in pan.

Whisk remaining 3 ingredients in medium bowl. Pour over sausage mixture. Heat and stir for 5 seconds. Reduce heat to medium-low. Cook, covered, for about 5 minutes until bottom is set.

Sprinkle cheese over top. Broil on centre rack in oven for about 5 minutes until top is set and golden (see Tip, below). Cuts into 4 wedges.

tip When baking or broiling food in a frying pan with a handle that isn't ovenproof, wrap the handle in foil and keep it to the front of the oven, away from the element.

Butter Chicken Curry

Absolutely delicious! Lean chicken is coated in a spice mix for maximum flavour.

Canola oil	1 tbsp.	15 mL
Curry powder	1 tbsp.	15 mL
Finely grated ginger root (or 3/4 tsp., 4 mL, ground ginger)	1 tbsp.	15 mL
Brown sugar, packed	1 tsp.	5 mL
Ground cumin	1/2 tsp.	2 mL
Salt	1/2 tsp.	2 mL
Boneless, skinless chicken breast halves, quartered	1 lb.	454 g
Butter	1 tsp.	5 mL
Canola oil	1 tsp.	5 mL
Finely chopped onion	1 1/2 cups	375 mL
Garlic cloves, minced (or 1/2 tsp., 2 mL, powder)	2	2
Tomato paste (see Tip, page 32)	3 tbsp.	50 mL
Curry powder	1 tsp.	5 mL
Brown sugar, packed	1/2 tsp.	2 mL
Ground cinnamon	1/4 tsp.	1 mL
Prepared chicken broth	1 cup	250 mL
Plain Balkan-style yogurt	1/2 cup	125 mL
Chopped fresh cilantro (optional)	1 tbsp.	15 mL

BEFORE: *1 serving:*
*436 Calories; **29.6 g Total Fat** (15.6 Sat);
726.7 mg Sodium*

AFTER: *1 serving:*
*243 Calories; **7 g Total Fat** (3.5 g Mono,
1.5 g Poly, 1.5 g Sat);
69 mg Cholesterol;
14 g Carbohydrate;
3 g Fibre; 30 g Protein;
577 mg Sodium*

Combine first 6 ingredients in medium bowl. Add chicken. Toss until coated. Place on greased baking sheet with sides. Cook in 450°F (230°C) oven for about 10 minutes until no longer pink inside.

Heat butter and second amount of canola oil in large frying pan on medium. Add onion and garlic. Cook for about 10 minutes, stirring often, until onion is softened and browned.

Add next 4 ingredients. Heat and stir for 1 minute. Add broth. Stir. Bring to a boil. Reduce heat to medium-low. Add chicken. Cook for about 5 minutes, stirring occasionally, until heated through. Remove from heat.

Stir in yogurt and cilantro. Serves 4.

Creamy Chicken Casserole

A classic chicken, broccoli and rice casserole that skips high-sodium canned soup in favour of a homemade creamy vegetable mixture.

All-purpose flour	3 tbsp.	50 mL
Milk	1 1/2 cups	375 mL
Boneless, skinless chicken breast halves, cut into 3/4 inch (2 cm) pieces	1 lb.	454 g
Sliced fresh white mushrooms	2 cups	500 mL
Chopped onion	1 cup	250 mL
Long-grain brown rice	1 cup	250 mL
Prepared chicken broth	1 cup	250 mL
Sliced celery	1 cup	250 mL
Dried rosemary, crushed	1/4 tsp.	1 mL
Dried thyme	1/4 tsp.	1 mL
Salt	1/4 tsp.	1 mL
Pepper	1/2 tsp.	2 mL
Small broccoli florets	2 cups	500 mL
Fine dry bread crumbs	1/2 cup	125 mL
Grated Parmesan cheese	1/2 cup	125 mL
Canola oil	1 tbsp.	15 mL

Whisk flour into milk in large bowl until smooth.

Add next 10 ingredients. Stir. Transfer to greased 9 x 13 inch (23 x 33 cm) baking dish. Cook, covered, in 375°F (190°C) oven for 45 minutes.

Add broccoli. Stir well. Cook, covered, for about 35 minutes until rice is tender.

Combine remaining 3 ingredients in small bowl. Sprinkle over top. Broil on centre rack for about 3 minutes until golden. Let stand, covered, for 10 minutes. Serves 6.

BEFORE: *1 serving: **581 Calories**; 27 g Total Fat (8 g Sat); 912 mg Sodium*

AFTER: *1 serving: **340 Calories**; 7 g Total Fat (2.5 g Mono, 1 g Poly, 2 g Sat); 53 mg Cholesterol; 42 g Carbohydrate; 3 g Fibre; 27 g Protein; 454 mg Sodium*

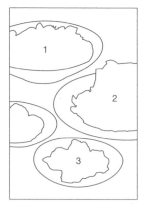

1. Barley Beef Stew, page 48
2. Beef Pot Pie, page 49
3. Sweet and Sour Meatballs, page 37

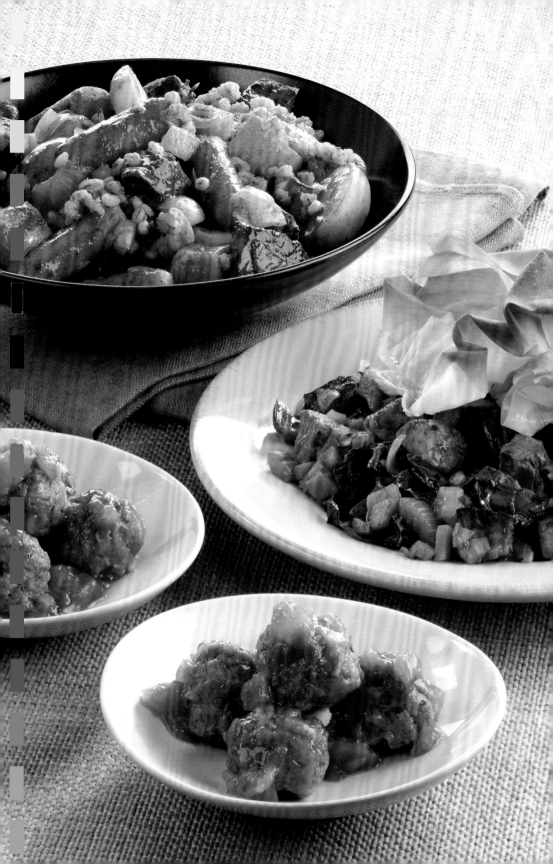

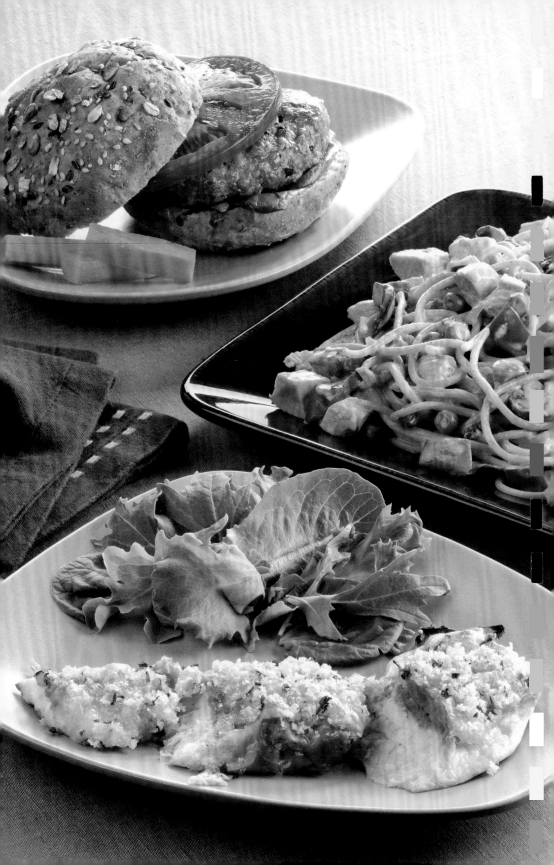

Tuscan Turkey Burgers

Lean turkey is a healthy alternative to beef in these burgers. The spinach, dressing and tomato toppings are so tasty that there's no need to load on any fattening condiments.

Egg whites (large)	2	2
Large flake rolled oats	3/4 cup	175 mL
Finely chopped fresh spinach leaves, lightly packed	1/3 cup	75 mL
Sun-dried tomato (or Italian) dressing	2 tbsp.	30 mL
Grated Parmesan cheese	1 tbsp.	15 mL
Pepper	1/4 tsp.	1 mL
Garlic powder	1/8 tsp.	0.5 mL
Lean ground turkey thigh	1 lb.	454 g
Cooking spray		
Fresh spinach leaves, lightly packed	1 cup	250 mL
Sun-dried tomato (or Italian) dressing	1 tbsp.	15 mL
Multi-grain (or whole-wheat) rolls, split	4	4
Large tomato, sliced	1	1

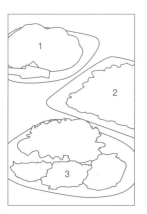

1. Tuscan Turkey Burgers, above
2. Turkey Tetrazzini, page 56
3. Cordon Bleu Chicken, page 57

Combine first 7 ingredients in medium bowl. Add turkey. Mix well. Divide into 4 equal portions. Shape into 4 inch (10 cm) diameter patties. Arrange on greased baking sheet with sides.

Spray with cooking spray. Broil on top rack in oven for about 5 minutes per side until internal temperature reaches 175°F (80°C).

Toss second amounts of spinach and dressing in small bowl. Arrange on bottom halves of rolls. Serve patties topped with tomato in rolls. Makes 4 burgers.

Pictured at left.

BEFORE: *1 burger: 593 Calories; 35.9 Total Fat (10 g Sat); **2 g Fibre**; 796 mg Sodium*

AFTER: *1 burger: 445 Calories; 13 g Total Fat (0.5 g Mono, 1.5 g Poly, 2 g Sat); 64 mg Cholesterol; 55 g Carbohydrate; **6 g Fibre**; 34 g Protein; 656 mg Sodium*

Turkey Tetrazzini

A lighter cream sauce reduces the total fat, while whole-wheat spaghetti and colourful vegetables add fibre.

Water	12 cups	3 L
Salt	1 1/2 tsp.	7 mL
Whole-wheat spaghetti, broken in half	8 oz.	225 g
Canola oil	2 tsp.	10 mL
Sliced fresh brown (or white) mushrooms	2 cups	500 mL
Chopped onion	1 cup	250 mL
Diced red pepper	1 cup	250 mL
Prepared chicken broth	1 1/2 cups	375 mL
Dry (or alcohol-free) white wine	1/4 cup	60 mL
Pepper	1/4 tsp.	1 mL
Diced cooked turkey breast	2 cups	500 mL
Frozen peas, thawed	1 cup	250 mL
Block light cream cheese, softened	4 oz.	125 g
Light sour cream	1/2 cup	125 mL
Grated Parmesan cheese	1/4 cup	60 mL

BEFORE: *1 cup (250 mL): 301 Calories; **12 g Total Fat** (6.5 g Sat); 1.6 g Fibre; 593 mg Sodium*

AFTER: *1 cup (250 mL): 260 Calories; **6 g Total Fat** (1.5 g Mono, 1 g Poly, 2.5 g Sat); 38 mg Cholesterol; 32 g Carbohydrate; 4 g Fibre; 20 g Protein; 280 mg Sodium*

Combine water and salt in Dutch oven. Bring to a boil. Add pasta. Boil, uncovered, for 10 to 12 minutes, stirring occasionally, until tender but firm. Drain. Return to same pot. Cover to keep warm.

Heat canola oil in large frying pan on medium. Add mushrooms and onion. Cook for about 10 minutes, stirring often, until onion is softened. Add red pepper. Stir. Cook for 2 minutes.

Add next 3 ingredients. Bring to a boil.

Add next 4 ingredients. Stir. Cook for about 5 minutes, stirring occasionally, until heated through. Add pasta. Toss.

Sprinkle Parmesan cheese over top. Stir. Makes about 7 1/2 cups (1.9 L).

Pictured on page 54.

Cordon Bleu Chicken

Rich and decadent, this is perfect for entertaining! Splitting the chicken breasts makes for much healthier portion sizes than classic Cordon Bleu recipes.

Boneless, skinless chicken breast halves (4 – 6 oz., 113 – 170 g, each)	4	4
Garlic powder	1/2 tsp.	2 mL
Pepper	1/4 tsp.	1 mL
Shaved lean deli ham	5 oz.	140 g
Grated Swiss cheese	1 cup	250 mL
Panko (or fine dry) bread crumbs	1/2 cup	125 mL
Canola oil	1 tbsp.	15 mL
Chopped fresh parsley	1 tbsp.	15 mL

BEFORE: *1 piece:*
***425 Calories**; 23.9 g Total Fat (8.2 g Sat); 1245 mg Sodium*

AFTER: *1 piece:*
***210 Calories**; 8 g Total Fat (1.5 g Mono, 0.5 g Poly, 3.5 g Sat); 75 mg Cholesterol; 4 g Carbohydrate; 0 g Fibre; 28 g Protein; 321 mg Sodium*

Cut each chicken breast in half horizontally. Place 1 chicken piece between 2 sheets of plastic wrap. Pound with mallet or rolling pin to 1/4 inch (6 mm) thickness. Repeat with remaining chicken.

Sprinkle garlic powder and pepper on both sides of chicken. Arrange on greased baking sheet with sides.

Arrange ham over chicken. Sprinkle with cheese.

Combine remaining 3 ingredients in small bowl. Sprinkle over cheese. Cook in 375°F (190°C) oven for about 25 minutes until internal temperature reaches 170°F (77°C). Makes 8 pieces.

Pictured on page 54.

Paré Pointer

About the only person who really wants to be down and out is an astronaut.

Turkey Cannelloni

Low-fat ground turkey is a healthy filling for cannelloni, and apple is a fresh and unexpected addition.

Canola oil	2 tsp.	10 mL
Chopped onion	2 cups	500 mL
Finely chopped fennel bulb (white part only)	2 cups	500 mL
Italian seasoning	1 tbsp.	15 mL
Dried crushed chilies	1 tsp.	5 mL
Salt	1/2 tsp.	2 mL
Pepper	1/4 tsp.	1 mL
Chopped fresh spinach leaves, lightly packed	3 cups	750 mL
Lean ground turkey thigh	1/2 lb.	225 g
Finely chopped peeled tart apple (such as Granny Smith)	1 cup	250 mL
Large flake rolled oats	1/2 cup	125 mL
Can of diced tomatoes (with juice)	28 oz.	796 mL
Water	1/2 cup	125 mL
Tomato paste (see Tip, page 32)	3 tbsp.	50 mL
Oven-ready cannelloni shells	20	20
Grated Parmesan cheese	1 cup	250 mL

BEFORE: *1 serving:*
734 Calories; 43 g Total Fat
*(**21 g Sat**); 1409 mg Sodium*

AFTER: *1 serving:*
319 Calories; 8 g Total Fat
(2 g Mono, 1 g Poly,
***2 g Sat**);*
30 mg Cholesterol;
45 g Carbohydrate;
6 g Fibre; 19 g Protein;
900 mg Sodium

Heat canola oil in large frying pan on medium. Add next 6 ingredients. Cook for about 10 minutes, stirring occasionally, until onion is softened. Add spinach. Heat and stir until just wilted. Remove from heat. Carefully process onion mixture in blender or food processor until finely chopped (see Safety Tip). Transfer to large bowl.

Add next 3 ingredients. Mix well. Spoon into large resealable freezer bag with corner snipped off.

Combine next 3 ingredients in medium bowl. Spread 1 cup (250 mL) tomato mixture in bottom of greased 9 x 13 inch (23 x 33 cm) baking dish.

(continued on next page)

Chicken & Turkey

Pipe turkey mixture into pasta shells. Arrange in single layer over tomato mixture in baking dish. Pour remaining tomato mixture over filled shells. Bake, covered, in 350°F (175°C) oven for about 50 minutes until turkey is no longer pink. Sprinkle with cheese. Bake, uncovered, for about 5 minutes until cheese is bubbling. Serves 6.

Safety Tip: Follow manufacturer's instructions for processing hot liquids.

Smoky Turkey Burritos

Easy to prepare. Tomato and coleslaw are a nice, light contrast to the bean and turkey mixture. Barbecue sauce adds a smoky, slightly sweet touch.

Canola oil	2 tsp.	10 mL
Extra-lean ground turkey breast	3/4 lb.	340 g
Chopped onion	1 cup	250 mL
Can of black beans, rinsed and drained, coarsely mashed	19 oz.	540 mL
Diced red pepper	1 cup	250 mL
Hickory barbecue sauce	1/4 cup	60 mL
Dried crushed chilies	1/2 tsp.	2 mL
Pepper	1/4 tsp.	1 mL
Diced seeded tomato	1 cup	250 mL
Coleslaw mix	2 cups	500 mL
Whole-wheat flour tortillas (10 inch, 25 cm, diameter)	6	6
Grated jalapeño Monterey Jack cheese	3/4 cup	175 mL

BEFORE: *1 wrap:*
644 Calories; **34 g Total Fat** *(11 g Sat);*
1727 mg Sodium

AFTER: *1 wrap:*
406 Calories; **10 g Total Fat** *(1 g Mono, 0.5 g Poly, 3.5 g Sat);*
40 mg Cholesterol;
53 g Carbohydrate;
10 g Fibre; 26 g Protein;
848 mg Sodium

Heat canola oil in large frying pan on medium. Add turkey and onion. Scramble-fry for about 8 minutes until turkey is no longer pink.

Add next 5 ingredients. Cook for about 5 minutes, stirring occasionally, until heated through. Remove from heat. Stir in tomato.

Scatter coleslaw along centre of tortillas. Spoon turkey mixture over coleslaw. Sprinkle cheese over turkey mixture. Fold sides over filling. Roll up tightly from bottom to enclose filling. Makes 6 wraps.

Spring Chicken Pot Pie

Using only a top crust for this hearty pot pie cuts way back on fat and calories.
To make this recipe gluten-free, use gluten-free chicken broth.

Canola oil	2 tsp.	10 mL
Boneless, skinless chicken breast halves, cut into 3/4 inch (2 cm) pieces	3/4 lb.	340 g
Sliced leek (white part only)	1 1/2 cups	375 mL
Diced unpeeled potato	1 cup	250 mL
Garlic cloves, minced (or 1/2 tsp., 2 mL, powder)	2	2
Salt	1/8 tsp.	0.5 mL
Pepper	1/4 tsp.	1 mL
Prepared chicken broth	1 1/2 cups	375 mL
Cornstarch	2 tbsp.	30 mL
Chopped trimmed asparagus	1 cup	250 mL
Frozen peas, thawed	1 cup	250 mL
Prepared chicken broth	3 cups	750 mL
Yellow cornmeal	1 cup	250 mL
Chopped green onion (green part only)	1 tbsp.	15 mL
Chopped fresh dill (or 3/4 tsp., 4 mL, dried)	1 tbsp.	15 mL

BEFORE: *1 serving:*
*875 Calories; **54 g Total Fat** (26 g Sat); 1463 Sodium*

AFTER: *1 serving:*
*378 Calories; **3.5 g Total Fat** (1.5 g Mono, 1 g Poly, 0.5 g Sat);*
49 mg Cholesterol;
57 g Carbohydrate;
5 g Fibre; 26 g Protein;
806 mg Sodium

Heat canola oil in large saucepan on medium. Add next 6 ingredients. Cook for about 10 minutes, stirring often, until chicken is no longer pink and potato is tender.

Stir first amount of broth into cornstarch in small bowl. Add to chicken mixture. Bring to a boil. Cook for 2 minutes, stirring occasionally. Add asparagus and peas. Stir. Transfer to greased 8 x 8 inch (20 x 20 cm) baking dish.

Bring second amount of broth to a boil in medium saucepan. Add cornmeal. Heat and stir for about 5 minutes until mixture thickens and pulls away from side of pan. Stir in green onion and dill. Pour evenly over chicken mixture. Bake in 375°F (190°C) oven for about 35 minutes until bubbling and topping is set. Serves 4.

Turkey Jambalaya

Feel the heat! You can dial the heat of this Cajun-inspired dish up or down by adjusting the amount of hot sauce.

Canola oil	1 tbsp.	15 mL
Boneless, skinless turkey thighs, cut into 1 inch (2.5 cm) pieces	1 1/2 lbs.	680 g
Uncooked Chorizo (or hot Italian) sausages	1/2 lb.	225 g
Chopped celery	1 cup	250 mL
Chopped green pepper	1 cup	250 mL
Chopped onion	1 cup	250 mL
Garlic cloves, minced (or 1/2 tsp., 2 mL, powder)	2	2
Long-grain white rice	1 cup	250 mL
Can of diced tomatoes (with juice)	28 oz.	796 mL
Water	2 cups	500 mL
Tomato paste (see Tip, page 32)	3 tbsp.	50 mL
Worcestershire sauce	1 tbsp.	15 mL
Cajun seasoning	1 1/2 tsp.	7 mL
Louisiana hot sauce	1 tsp.	5 mL

BEFORE: *1 cup (250 mL):*
338 Calories; *17.9 Total Fat (6.2 g Sat); 701 mg Sodium*

AFTER: *1 cup (250 mL):*
180 Calories; *8 g Total Fat (1.5 g Mono, 1 g Poly, 2 g Sat); 49 mg Cholesterol; 15 g Carbohydrate; 1 g Fibre; 13 g Protein; 450 mg Sodium*

Heat canola oil in Dutch oven on medium-high. Add turkey. Cook for about 5 minutes, stirring occasionally, until no longer pink. Remove to plate. Cover to keep warm.

Add sausages to same pot. Cook for about 4 minutes, turning occasionally, until browned on all sides. Remove to cutting board. Cut into 1/2 inch (12 mm) slices. Cover to keep warm.

Add next 4 ingredients to same pot. Reduce heat to medium. Cook for about 5 minutes, stirring often, until onion is softened. Add rice. Stir.

Add remaining 6 ingredients. Stir. Bring to a boil. Add turkey and sausage. Stir. Reduce heat to medium-low. Simmer, covered, for about 20 minutes, without stirring, until rice is tender. Remove from heat. Let stand, covered, for 5 minutes. Stir. Makes about 15 cups (3.75 L).

Chicken Biscuit Stew

Not only is this recipe lower in calories, fat and sodium, but it's also high in fibre and piles on the vegetables. You definitely can't go wrong with that!

Canola oil	1 tsp.	5 mL
Boneless, skinless chicken thighs, halved	2 lbs.	900 g
All-purpose flour	3 tbsp.	50 mL
Garlic powder	1/2 tsp.	2 mL
Dried dillweed	1/2 tsp.	2 mL
Salt	1/8 tsp.	0.5 mL
Pepper	1/4 tsp.	1 mL
Prepared chicken broth	1 1/2 cups	375 mL
Chopped fresh (or frozen cut) green beans	1 cup	250 mL
Chopped onion	1 cup	250 mL
Chopped unpeeled potato	1 cup	250 mL
Sliced carrot	1 cup	250 mL
Sliced celery	1 cup	250 mL
CHEDDAR RANCH BISCUITS		
Whole-wheat flour	1 1/2 cups	375 mL
Grated sharp Cheddar cheese	2/3 cup	150 mL
Baking powder	2 tsp.	10 mL
Cold butter	1 tbsp.	15 mL
Fat-free ranch dressing	3/4 cup	175 mL
Canola oil	1 tbsp.	15 mL

BEFORE: *1 serving:*
575 Calories; *22.1 g Total Fat (4.8 g Sat); 1324 mg Sodium*

AFTER: *1 serving:*
360 Calories; *11 g Total Fat (4 g Mono, 2 g Poly, 4 g Sat); 106 mg Cholesterol; 36 g Carbohydrate; 5 g Fibre; 29 g Protein; 660 mg Sodium*

Heat canola oil in large frying pan on medium-high. Add chicken. Cook for about 10 minutes, stirring occasionally, until browned.

Add next 5 ingredients. Heat and stir for 1 minute. Slowly add broth, stirring constantly until smooth. Transfer chicken mixture to greased 3 quart (3 L) casserole.

Add remaining 5 ingredients. Stir. Bake, covered, in 375°F (190°C) oven for about 1 hour until potato and carrot are tender. Stir.

Cheddar Ranch Biscuits: Combine first 3 ingredients in medium bowl. Cut in butter until mixture resembles coarse crumbs.

(continued on next page)

Add dressing and canola oil. Stir until just moistened. Drop batter onto hot chicken mixture in 8 mounds, using about 1/4 cup (60 mL) for each. Bake, uncovered, for about 20 minutes until wooden pick inserted in centre of biscuit comes out clean. Serves 8.

Oven-Fried Chicken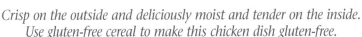

Crisp on the outside and deliciously moist and tender on the inside.
Use gluten-free cereal to make this chicken dish gluten-free.

Crisp rice cereal	4 cups	1 L
Sesame seeds	2 tbsp.	30 mL
Egg white (large), fork beaten	1	1
1% buttermilk	1/3 cup	75 mL
Dijon mustard	2 tsp.	10 mL
Garlic powder	1/4 tsp.	1 mL
Paprika	1/4 tsp.	1 mL
Salt	1/2 tsp	2 mL
Pepper	1/4 tsp.	1 mL
Boneless, skinless chicken breast halves (4 – 6 oz., 113 – 170 g, each)	6	6
Cornstarch	3 tbsp.	50 mL
Cooking spray		

BEFORE: *1 piece:*
531 Calories; **32.9 g Total Fat** *(4.8 g Sat);*
1372 mg Sodium

AFTER: *1 piece:*
220 Calories; **2 g Total Fat** *(0 g Mono, 0 g Poly, 0.5 g Sat);*
97 mg Cholesterol;
7 g Carbohydrate;
1 g Fibre; 40 g Protein;
280 mg Sodium

Process cereal and sesame seeds in food processor until mixture resembles coarse crumbs. Transfer to large shallow dish.

Whisk next 7 ingredients in medium bowl until smooth.

Press chicken in cornstarch on large plate until coated on both sides. Lightly brush off any excess. Dip into buttermilk mixture. Press in cereal mixture until coated. Place on well-greased rack set in foil-lined baking sheet. Discard any excess cornstarch, egg mixture and cereal mixture.

Spray chicken with cooking spray. Cook in 425°F (220°C) oven for about 30 minutes until golden and internal temperature reaches 170°F (77°C). Makes 6 pieces.

Corn Crab Cakes

Shrimp and celery are lovely accents in these low-fat, sodium-reduced crab cakes.

Egg white (large)	1	1
Fat-free ranch dressing	3 tbsp.	50 mL
Dried crushed chilies	1/4 tsp.	1 mL
Salt	1/8 tsp.	0.5 mL
Pepper	1/4 tsp.	1 mL
Cans of crabmeat (4 1/2 oz., 120 g, each), drained, cartilage removed, flaked	2	2
Uncooked shrimp (peeled and deveined), finely chopped	1/2 lb.	225 g
Fresh (or frozen, thawed) kernel corn, chopped	1 cup	250 mL
Yellow cornmeal	3/4 cup	175 mL
Finely chopped celery	1/4 cup	60 mL
Finely chopped green onion	1/4 cup	60 mL
Finely chopped fresh parsley (or 3/4 tsp., 4 mL, flakes)	1 tbsp.	15 mL
Canola oil	2 tbsp.	30 mL

BEFORE: *1 crab cake:*
270 Calories; **15.5 g Total Fat** *(2.3 g Sat);*
517 mg Sodium

AFTER: *1 crab cake:*
162 Calories; **4 g Total Fat** *(2 g Mono, 1 g Poly, 0 g Sat);*
62 mg Cholesterol;
19 g Carbohydrate;
1 g Fibre; 11 g Protein;
269 mg Sodium

Whisk first 5 ingredients in medium bowl.

Add next 7 ingredients. Mix well. Divide into 8 equal portions. Shape into 1/2 inch (12 mm) thick cakes. Chill, covered, for 30 minutes.

Heat 1 tbsp. (15 mL) canola oil in large frying pan on medium (see Note). Cook 4 crab cakes for about 5 minutes per side until browned. Repeat with remaining canola oil and crab cakes. Makes 8 crab cakes.

Note: To reduce fat even more, crab cakes can be baked in the oven. Arrange crab cakes on greased baking sheet with sides. Bake in 375°F (190°C) oven for about 10 minutes per side until browned.

Tuna Vegetable Casserole

Bring back childhood memories with this healthy new take on a classic. The mixed vegetables add interest and are good for you, too. You can substitute the same volume of any small whole-wheat pasta for the noodles.

Water	8 cups	2 L
Salt	1 tsp.	5 mL
Whole-wheat egg noodles	4 cups	1 L
Butter	1 tbsp.	15 mL
Chopped fresh white mushrooms	1 cup	250 mL
Finely chopped onion	1 cup	250 mL
All-purpose flour	3 tbsp.	50 mL
Salt	1/4 tsp.	1 mL
Pepper	1/4 tsp.	1 mL
Milk	3 cups	750 mL
Cans of flaked light tuna in water, drained (6 oz., 170 g, each)	2	2
Frozen mixed vegetables, thawed	2 cups	500 mL
Fresh whole-wheat bread crumbs (about 2 bread slices)	1 cup	250 mL
Grated Parmesan cheese	1/2 cup	125 mL

BEFORE: *1 serving:*
*313 Calories; **13 g Total Fat** (5.3 g Sat); 1 g Fibre; 722 mg Sodium*

AFTER: *1 serving:*
*320 Calories; **7 g Total Fat** (1 g Mono, 0 g Poly, 3.5 g Sat); 50 mg Cholesterol; 41 g Carbohydrate; 4 g Fibre; 25 g Protein; 527 mg Sodium*

Combine water and salt in large saucepan. Bring to a boil. Add noodles. Boil, uncovered, for about 5 minutes, stirring occasionally, until tender but firm. Drain. Return to same pot. Cover to keep warm.

Melt butter in large saucepan on medium. Add mushrooms and onion. Cook for about 10 minutes, stirring often, until mushrooms start to brown. Add next 3 ingredients. Heat and stir for 1 minute.

Slowly add milk, stirring constantly until smooth. Cook for about 8 minutes, stirring often, until boiling and thickened. Pour over noodles.

Add tuna and vegetables. Mix well. Transfer to greased 2 quart (2 L) casserole.

Combine bread crumbs and cheese in small bowl. Sprinkle over noodle mixture. Bake, uncovered, in 350°F (175°C) oven for about 30 minutes until bubbling and topping is golden brown. Serves 6.

Vodka Linguine and Clams

A decadent pasta dish that's definitely worthy of a special occasion!
Celebrate in style and serve with a glass of red wine.

Prepared chicken broth	2 cups	500 mL
Package of dried mixed mushrooms	1/2 oz.	14 g
Olive oil	1 tsp.	5 mL
Chopped red onion	1 cup	250 mL
Garlic cloves, minced	3	3
Reserved clam liquid	1 cup	250 mL
Vodka	1/2 cup	125 mL
Pepper	1/4 tsp.	1 mL
Cans of whole baby clams (5 oz., 142 g, each), drained and liquid reserved	2	2
Block light cream cheese, cut up	4 oz.	125 g
Lemon juice	1 tbsp.	15 mL
Water	12 cups	3 L
Salt	1 1/2 tsp.	7 mL
Linguine	12 oz.	340 g
Grated Parmesan cheese	1/2 cup	125 mL
Chopped fresh parsley	3 tbsp.	50 mL

BEFORE: *1 cup (250 mL):*
421 Calories, **18 g Total**
Fat *(10 g Sat);*
547 mg Sodium

AFTER: *1 cup (250 mL):*
319 Calories; **7 g Total**
Fat *(1 g Mono, 0 g Poly,*
3 g Sat); 40 mg Cholesterol;
40 g Carbohydrate;
2 g Fibre; 16 g Protein;
500 mg Sodium

Bring broth to a boil in small saucepan. Add mushrooms. Remove from heat. Let stand, covered, for 10 minutes. Remove mushrooms. Strain mushroom liquid through double layer of cheesecloth into small bowl. Chop mushrooms.

Heat olive oil in large frying pan on medium. Add onion and garlic. Cook for about 5 minutes, stirring often, until onion is softened.

Add next 3 ingredients, mushrooms and mushroom liquid. Stir. Bring to a boil. Reduce heat to medium-low. Simmer, uncovered, for 15 minutes.

Add next 3 ingredients. Heat and stir until cream cheese is melted.

(continued on next page)

Combine water and salt in Dutch oven. Bring to a boil. Add pasta. Boil, uncovered, for 9 to 11 minutes, stirring occasionally, until tender but firm. Drain. Add to clam mixture.

Add Parmesan cheese and parsley. Toss. Makes about 7 1/2 cups (1.9 L).

Oven-Fried Fish

It's so easy to make fish and chips at home with the help of this handy fish recipe. And so quick, too! Try with the Triple-Chili Oven Fries on page 115.

All-purpose flour	1/4 cup	60 mL
Cajun seasoning	1/2 tsp.	2 mL
Cayenne pepper	1/8 tsp.	0.5 mL
Egg whites (large)	2	2
Crushed cornflakes cereal	3/4 cup	175 mL
Seasoned salt	1/2 tsp.	2 mL
Haddock fillets, any small bones removed	1 lb.	454 g
Cooking spray		

BEFORE: *1 serving:*
303 Calories; **13.9 g Total Fat** *(1.8 g Sat);*
884 mg Sodium

AFTER: *1 serving:*
177 Calories; **1 g Total Fat** *(0 g Mono, 0 g Poly, 0 g Sat); 65 mg Cholesterol; 15 g Carbohydrate; 0 g Fibre; 25 g Protein; 367 mg Sodium*

Combine first 3 ingredients on large plate.

Beat egg white in small shallow bowl.

Combine cereal and seasoned salt in medium shallow bowl.

Press fillets, 1 at a time, in flour mixture. Dip into egg. Press into crumb mixture until coated. Arrange on greased baking sheet. Discard any remaining flour mixture, egg and crumb mixture.

Spray fish with cooking spray. Bake in 450°F (230°C) oven for 8 to 9 minutes until fish flakes easily when tested with fork. Serves 4.

Paré Pointer

We'd have good heads on our shoulders if it wasn't for our necks.

Lemon Dill Salmon Cakes

Cooking salmon cakes under the broiler is healthier than frying, since you don't have to add any additional oil. Packed with vegetables that add lots of nutrients.

Canned navy beans, rinsed and drained	1 cup	250 mL
Chopped carrot	1/2 cup	125 mL
Chopped celery	1/2 cup	125 mL
Chopped onion	1/2 cup	125 mL
Chopped fresh parsley (or 1 tbsp., 15 mL, flakes)	1/4 cup	60 mL
Dried dillweed	1 tbsp.	15 mL
Lemon juice	1 tbsp.	15 mL
Grated lemon zest (see Tip, page 151)	1 tsp.	5 mL
Salt	1/2 tsp.	2 mL
Pepper	1/2 tsp.	2 mL
Salmon fillet, skin and any small bones removed, coarsely chopped	1 lb.	454 g
Yellow cornmeal	1/4 cup	60 mL
Cooking spray		

BEFORE: *1 salmon cake:*
165 Calories; *11 g Total Fat (2 g Sat); 402 mg Sodium*

AFTER: *1 salmon cake:*
86 Calories; *2 g Total Fat (1 g Mono, 1 g Poly, 0 g Sat); 19 mg Cholesterol; 7 g Carbohydrate; 1 g Fibre; 8 g Protein; 148 mg Sodium*

Process first 10 ingredients in food processor until coarsely chopped.

Add salmon. Process until salmon is coarsely ground and mixture comes together. Transfer to medium bowl.

Add cornmeal. Mix well. Using about 1/4 cup (60 mL) for each, shape into 2 inch (5 cm) cakes. Arrange on greased baking sheet with sides.

Spray patties with cooking spray. Broil on top rack in oven for about 3 minutes per side until internal temperature reaches 160°F (71°C). Makes about 13 salmon cakes.

Pictured on page 71.

Lemon Ginger Seafood Stir-Fry

This punchy, lemony sauce is much healthier than pre-made stir-fry sauces and goes well with the slightly sweet red pepper and snap peas. Serve with brown basmati rice.

Prepared vegetable broth	1 cup	250 mL
Cornstarch	2 tbsp.	30 mL
Lemon juice	2 tbsp.	30 mL
Brown sugar, packed	1 tbsp.	15 mL
Finely grated ginger root (or 3/4 tsp., 4 mL, ground ginger)	1 tbsp.	15 mL
Soy sauce	1 tbsp.	15 mL
Sesame oil (for flavour)	1 tsp.	5 mL
Garlic cloves, minced (or 1/2 tsp., 2 mL, powder)	2	2
Grated lemon zest (see Tip, page 151)	1/2 tsp.	2 mL
Canola oil	1 tsp.	5 mL
Sugar snap peas, trimmed	2 cups	500 mL
Thinly sliced onion	1 cup	250 mL
Thinly sliced red pepper	1 cup	250 mL
Sliced green onion (1 inch, 2.5 cm, pieces)	1/4 cup	60 mL
Halibut fillet, skin and any small bones removed, cut into bite-sized pieces	1/2 lb.	225 g
Small bay scallops	1/2 lb.	225 g

BEFORE: *1 cup (250 mL):*
260 Calories; 8 g Total Fat (0 g Sat); **2588 mg Sodium**

AFTER: *1 cup (250 mL):*
174 Calories; 3 g Total Fat (1.5 g Mono, 1 g Poly, 0 g Sat); 29 mg Cholesterol; 17 g Carbohydrate; 2 g Fibre; 19 g Protein; **444 mg Sodium**

Stir first 9 ingredients in small bowl.

Heat canola oil in large frying pan or wok on medium-high until very hot. Add next 4 ingredients. Stir-fry for about 2 minutes until vegetables are tender-crisp. Stir broth mixture. Add to vegetable mixture. Heat and stir until boiling and slightly thickened.

Add fish and scallops. Cook for about 3 minutes, stirring occasionally, until fish flakes easily when tested with fork and scallops turn opaque. Makes about 5 cups (1.25 L).

Pictured on page 71.

Coconut Shrimp

Instead of serving these shrimp with a high-sodium sauce, we've added a curry spice mix directly to the shrimp, delivering plenty of flavour with way less fat!

Cornstarch	3 tbsp.	50 mL
Hot curry powder (optional)	1 tsp.	5 mL
Salt	1/2 tsp.	2 mL
Pepper	1/4 tsp.	1 mL
Uncooked extra-large shrimp (peeled and deveined), blotted dry	1 lb.	454 g
Egg whites (large)	2	2
Medium unsweetened coconut	1 cup	250 mL

Cooking spray

Combine first 4 ingredients in large bowl. Add shrimp. Toss until coated. Discard any remaining cornstarch mixture.

Beat egg whites in small shallow bowl until frothy. Dip shrimp, 1 at a time, into egg whites until coated. Press both sides of shrimp into coconut on large plate. Place on greased baking sheet with sides.

Spray shrimp with cooking spray. Cook in 425°F (220°C) oven for about 5 minutes per side until shrimp turn pink. Makes about 30 coconut shrimp.

Pictured at right.

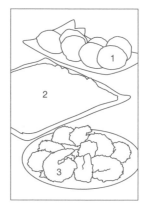

1. Lemon Dill Salmon Cakes, page 68
2. Lemon Ginger Seafood Stir-Fry, page 69
3. Coconut Shrimp, above

BEFORE: *2 shrimp: 230 Calories;* ***15.4 g Total Fat*** *(10 g Sat); 316 mg Sodium*

AFTER: *2 shrimp: 80 Calories;* ***4.5 g Total Fat*** *(0 g Mono, 0 g Poly, 4 g Sat); 46 mg Cholesterol; 3 g Carbohydrate; 1 g Fibre; 7 g Protein; 94 mg Sodium*

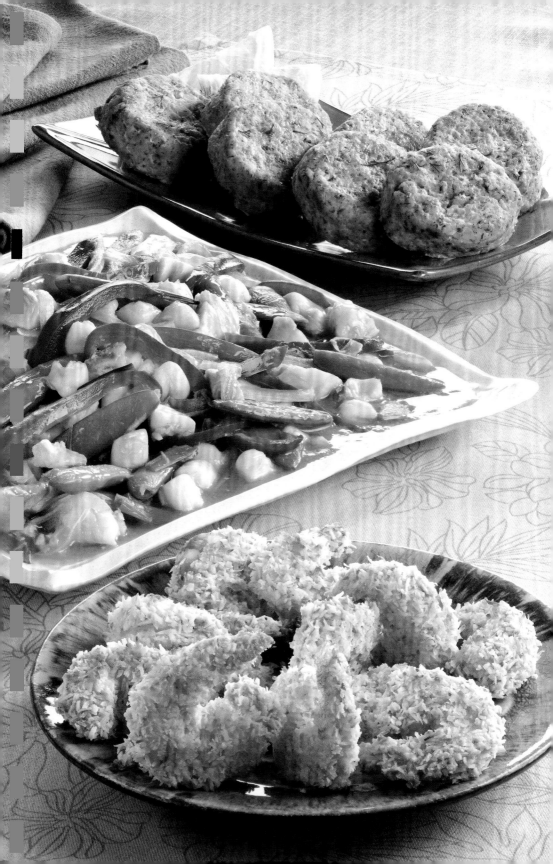

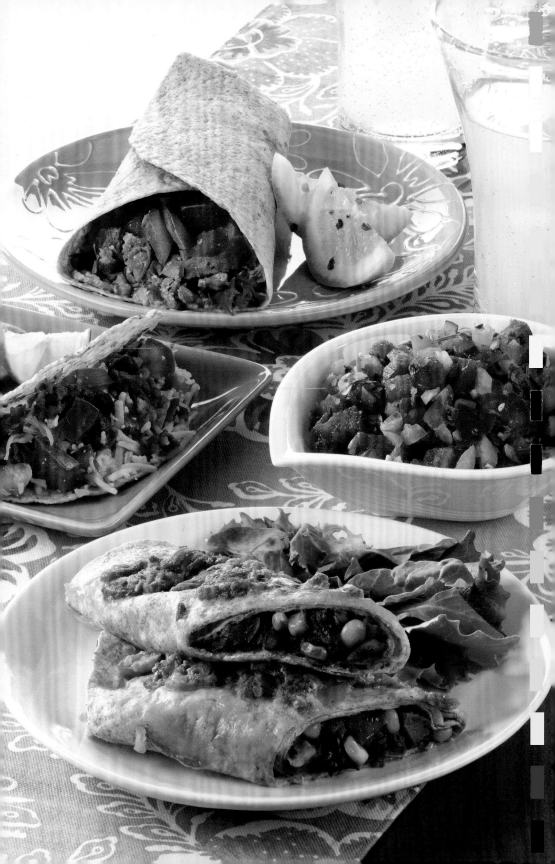

FLT Tacos

A fresh, healthy spin on fish tacos. Salmon and avocado abound in healthy fats and nutrients. A very satisfying meal.

Salmon fillets, skin and any small bones removed	3/4 lb.	340 g
Salt	1/4 tsp.	1 mL
Pepper	1/8 tsp.	0.5 mL
Mashed avocado	1 cup	250 mL
Chopped fresh chives	1 tbsp.	15 mL
Finely chopped fresh jalapeño pepper (see Tip, page 13)	1 tbsp.	15 mL
Lemon juice	1 tbsp.	15 mL
Sour cream	1 tbsp.	15 mL
Whole-wheat flour tortillas (10 inch, 25 cm, diameter)	4	4
Spring mix lettuce, lightly packed	2 cups	500 mL
Diced seeded tomato	2/3 cup	150 mL

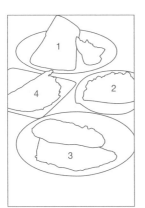

Arrange fillets on greased baking sheet with sides. Sprinkle with salt and pepper. Cook in 400°F (205°C) oven for about 10 minutes until fish flakes easily when tested with fork. Break into small chunks.

Combine next 5 ingredients in small bowl.

Spread avocado mixture over tortillas. Scatter lettuce mix, salmon and tomato, in order given, over avocado mixture. Fold bottom over filling. Fold sides over. Makes 4 soft tacos.

Pictured at left and on back cover.

1. FLT Tacos, above
2. Simply Fresh Salsa, page 120
3. Veggie Bean Enchiladas, page 94
4. Salsa Beef Tacos, page 34

Props: Moderno

BEFORE: *1 taco: 720 Calories; 55 g Total Fat (6 g Sat); 6 g Fibre; 1483 mg Sodium*

AFTER: *1 taco: 428 Calories; 23 g Total Fat (13 g Mono, 4.5 g Poly, 3.5 g Sat); 56 mg Cholesterol; 33 g Carbohydrate; 10 g Fibre; 27 g Protein; 676 mg Sodium*

Creamy Seafood Medley

Finally—proof that you can have a deliciously creamy dish that's still low in fat and calories! Try serving over pasta, noodles or potatoes.

Olive oil	1 tbsp.	15 mL
Thinly sliced leek (white part only)	2 cups	500 mL
Chopped fennel	1 cup	250 mL
Garlic cloves, minced (or 1/2 tsp., 2 mL, powder)	2	2
Dried basil	1/2 tsp.	2 mL
Salt	1/4 tsp.	1 mL
Pepper	1/4 tsp.	1 mL
Dry (or alcohol-free) white wine	1/2 cup	125 mL
All-purpose flour	1/4 cup	60 mL
Milk	3 cups	750 mL
Halibut fillets, skin and any small bones removed, cut into bite-sized pieces	1/2 lb.	225 g
Small bay scallops	1/2 lb.	225 g
Uncooked medium shrimp (peeled and deveined)	1/2 lb.	225 g
Grated Asiago cheese	1/4 cup	60 mL
Chopped fresh parsley (or 3/4 tsp., 4 mL, flakes)	1 tbsp.	15 mL
Lemon juice	2 tsp.	10 mL

BEFORE: *1 cup (250 mL):*
632 Calories; 49 g Total Fat
*(**29 g Sat**); 529 mg Sodium*

AFTER: *1 cup (250 mL):*
270 Calories; 7 g Total Fat
(2 g Mono, 1 g Poly,
***2 g Sat**); 91 mg Cholesterol;*
19 g Carbohydrate;
2 g Fibre; 30 g Protein;
374 mg Sodium

Heat olive oil in large frying pan on medium. Add next 6 ingredients. Cook for about 10 minutes, stirring occasionally, until leek is softened. Add wine. Simmer for 2 minutes until liquid is evaporated.

Sprinkle with flour. Heat and stir for 2 minutes. Slowly add milk, stirring constantly. Heat and stir until boiling and thickened.

Add next 3 ingredients. Cook for about 5 minutes, stirring occasionally, until shrimp turn pink and scallops turn opaque. Remove from heat.

Add remaining 3 ingredients. Stir until cheese is melted. Makes about 6 cups (1.5 L).

Fiesta Fish Fingers

*Considerably leaner than the frozen deep-fried fish fingers you get from the store,
and tastier, too! Use gluten-free cereal to make this recipe gluten-free.*

Chili powder	1 tsp.	5 mL
Salt	1/4 tsp.	1 mL
Pepper	1/4 tsp.	1 mL
Crisp rice cereal, crushed into fine crumbs	3 cups	750 mL
Egg white (large)	1	1
Large egg	1	1
Haddock fillets, any small bones removed, cut crosswise into 1 inch (2.5 cm) strips	1 lb.	454 g

Cooking spray

BEFORE: *1 fish finger:*
*61 Calories; **2.8 g Total Fat**
(0.2 g Sat); 178 mg Sodium*

AFTER: *1 fish finger:*
*38 Calories; **0 g Total Fat**
(0 g Mono, 0 g Poly,
0 g Sat); 20 mg Cholesterol;
3 g Carbohydrate; 0 g Fibre;
5 g Protein; 92 mg Sodium*

Combine first 3 ingredients in medium shallow dish. Add 1/3 cup (75 mL) cereal. Mix well. Put remaining cereal in large plate.

Beat egg white and egg in separate medium shallow dish.

Press fish into chili powder mixture until coated. Dip into egg. Press into cereal until coated. Arrange on greased baking sheet with sides. Discard any remaining chili powder mixture, egg and cereal.

Spray fish with cooking spray. Bake in 450°F (230°C) oven for about 7 minutes until fish flakes easily when tested with fork. Makes about 20 fish fingers.

Paré Pointer

A cursor is someone whose computer has a virus.

Haddock Croquettes

Crisp and golden yet tender and delicious—these croquettes are a real crowd pleaser!

Peeled red potatoes, cut up	1/2 lb.	225 g
Haddock fillets, any small bones removed	1/2 lb.	225 g
Milk	3/4 cup	175 mL
Canola oil	1 tsp.	5 mL
Diced onion	1/3 cup	75 mL
Diced red pepper	1/3 cup	75 mL
Large egg, fork-beaten	1	1
Paprika	1/2 tsp.	2 mL
Salt	3/4 tsp.	4 mL
Pepper	1/4 tsp.	1 mL
Cayenne pepper (optional)	1/8 tsp.	0.5 mL
All-purpose flour	2 tbsp.	30 mL
Large egg, fork-beaten	1	1
Fine dry bread crumbs	1/3 cup	75 mL
Canola oil	1 cup	250 mL

BEFORE: *1 croquette:*
252 Calories; 11.2 g Total Fat (2.4 g Sat); 535.3 mg Sodium

AFTER: *1 croquette:*
107 Calories; 4.2 g Total Fat (1.7 g Mono, 0.9 g Poly, 0.5 g Sat); 56 mg Cholesterol; 10 g Carbohydrate; 1 g Fibre; 8 g Protein; 340 mg Sodium

Pour water into small saucepan until about 1 inch (2.5 cm) deep. Add potato. Cover. Bring to a boil. Reduce heat to medium. Boil for 12 to 15 minutes until tender. Drain. Mash. Transfer to large bowl.

Put fillets and milk into same small saucepan. Bring to a boil. Reduce heat to medium-low. Simmer for about 5 minutes until fish flakes easily when tested with fork. Drain. Flake fillets with fork. Add to mashed potato. Stir.

Heat first amount of canola oil in medium frying pan on medium. Add onion and red pepper. Cook for about 5 minutes, stirring often, until onion is softened. Add to potato mixture. Stir.

Combine next 5 ingredients in small bowl. Add to potato mixture. Stir until well combined. Shape into eight 2 inch (5 cm) logs.

(continued on next page)

Measure flour into medium shallow dish. Beat egg in separate medium shallow dish. Measure bread crumbs onto large plate. Roll logs in flour until coated. Dip into egg. Roll logs in bread crumbs until coated. Discard any remaining flour, egg and bread crumbs.

Heat second amount of canola oil in same medium frying pan on medium-high until a bread cube turns brown in 1 minute (375°F, 190°C). Shallow-fry logs for about 2 minutes, turning occasionally, until browned on all sides. Remove to paper towels to drain. Makes 8 croquettes.

Tuna Melt Pizza

Combines the popular flavours of pizza and tuna melt sandwiches into a new family-friendly hit. Also good for lunch the next day.

Prebaked multi-grain (or whole-wheat) pizza crust (12 inch, 30 cm, diameter)	1	1
Alfredo pasta sauce	1/2 cup	125 mL
Can of chunk light tuna in water, drained	6 oz.	170 g
Finely chopped red onion	1/4 cup	60 mL
Diced red pepper	2/3 cup	150 mL
Finely chopped celery	1/3 cup	75 mL
Grated Swiss cheese	1 cup	250 mL
Diced seeded tomato	1/2 cup	125 mL
Chopped fresh parsley	1 tbsp.	15 mL

BEFORE: *1 wedge:* **342 Calories**; *20 g Total Fat (6 g Sat); 611 mg Sodium*

AFTER: *1 wedge:* **170 Calories**; *6 g Total Fat (0 g Mono, 0 g Poly, 3 g Sat); 24 mg Cholesterol; 18 g Carbohydrate; 2 g Fibre; 11 g Protein; 338 mg Sodium*

Place crust on ungreased 12 inch (30 cm) pizza pan.

Combine next 3 ingredients in small bowl. Spread over crust.

Scatter next 3 ingredients, in order given, over tuna mixture. Bake in 475°F (240°C) oven for about 15 minutes until crust is browned.

Sprinkle with tomato and parsley. Cuts into 8 wedges.

Pictured on page 107.

Two-Potato Sausage Hash

We've included a small amount of sausage to provide a classic sausage hash taste, but you could also use lean, low-sodium ham instead.

Canola oil	1/2 tsp.	2 mL
Pork tenderloin, trimmed of fat, cut into 1/2 inch (12 mm) cubes	3/4 lb.	340 g
Hot Italian sausage, casing removed	4 oz.	113 g
Chopped onion	2 cups	500 mL
Diced green pepper	2 cups	500 mL
Diced peeled orange-fleshed sweet potato	2 cups	500 mL
Diced unpeeled potato	2 cups	500 mL
Dried oregano	1/2 tsp.	2 mL
Dried thyme	1/2 tsp.	2 mL
Grated Asiago cheese	1 cup	250 mL

BEFORE: *1 serving:*
548 Calories; **40 g Total Fat** *(15 g Sat); 1253 mg Sodium*

AFTER: *1 serving:*
310 Calories; **13 g Total Fat** *(1 g Mono, 0 g Poly, 5 g Sat); 60 mg Cholesterol; 25 g Carbohydrate; 4 g Fibre; 22 g Protein; 398 mg Sodium*

Heat canola oil in large frying pan on medium. Add pork and sausage. Scramble-fry for about 10 minutes until no longer pink. Transfer to greased 9 x 13 inch (23 x 33 cm) pan.

Add next 6 ingredients to same frying pan. Cook for about 10 minutes, stirring occasionally, until potato starts to soften. Add to pork mixture. Stir. Bake, covered, in 400°F (205°C) oven for about 30 minutes until potato is tender. Remove cover.

Sprinkle cheese over top. Bake, uncovered, for about 5 minutes until cheese is melted. Serves 6.

Paré Pointer

While February can't March, April May.

Sweet and Sour Pork

Recreate your favourite fast-food take-out with this healthier version. Making your own sauce and stir-frying lean pork tenderloin greatly reduces fat and sodium.

Soy sauce	1 tbsp.	15 mL
Finely grated ginger root (or 1/2 tsp., 2 mL, ground ginger)	2 tsp.	10 mL
Garlic cloves, minced (or 1/2 tsp., 2 mL, powder)	2	2
Pork tenderloin, trimmed of fat and cut into 3/4 inch (2 cm) cubes	1 lb.	454 g
Prepared chicken broth	1 cup	250 mL
Apricot jam	1/4 cup	60 mL
Rice vinegar	1/4 cup	60 mL
Cornstarch	2 tbsp.	30 mL
Pepper	1/4 tsp.	1 mL
Canola oil	2 tsp.	10 mL
Frozen Oriental vegetable mix, thawed	6 cups	1.5 L

BEFORE: *1 cup (250 mL):*
363 Calories; **16 g Total**
Fat *(3 g Sat);*
918 mg Sodium

AFTER: *1 cup (250 mL):*
210 Calories; **4 g Total**
Fat *(2 g Mono, 0.5 g Poly,*
1 g Sat); 49 mg Cholesterol;
20 g Carbohydrate;
3 g Fibre; 22 g Protein;
339 mg Sodium

Stir first 3 ingredients in medium bowl. Add pork. Stir until coated. Chill, covered, for 30 minutes.

Stir next 5 ingredients until smooth.

Heat canola oil in large frying pan or wok on medium-high until very hot. Add pork mixture. Stir-fry for about 5 minutes until browned. Transfer to large plate. Cover to keep warm.

Add vegetable mixture to same frying pan. Stir-fry for 2 minutes. Stir broth mixture. Add to pan. Bring to a boil. Add pork. Cook for about 2 minutes, stirring often, until heated through. Makes about 5 1/2 cups (1.4 L).

Lamb Moussaka

What's the secret of this lower-fat makeover of the traditional Greek casserole?
Adding lean ground turkey to the lamb—and no one will ever guess the turkey
is there!

Large eggplant, sliced lengthwise (1/2 inch, 12 mm, thick)	1	1
Small zucchini (with peel), sliced lengthwise (1/2 inch, 12 mm, thick)	2	2
Olive oil	1 tsp.	5 mL
Lean ground lamb	3/4 lb.	340 g
Extra-lean ground turkey breast	1/2 lb.	225 g
Chopped onion	1 cup	250 mL
Diced carrot	1 cup	250 mL
Garlic cloves, minced (or 1/2 tsp., 2 mL, powder)	2	2
Dried oregano	1 tsp.	5 mL
Ground cinnamon	1 tsp.	5 mL
Salt	1/4 tsp.	1 mL
Pepper	1/2 tsp.	2 mL
Can of crushed tomatoes	28 oz.	796 mL
All-purpose flour	1/3 cup	75 mL
Milk	3 cups	750 mL
Crumbled feta cheese	1/2 cup	125 mL
Grated Parmesan cheese	1/2 cup	125 mL

BEFORE: *1 piece:*
650 Calories; *30.3 g Total Fat (13.9 g Sat); 1231 mg Sodium*

AFTER: *1 piece:*
301 Calories; *12 g Total Fat (1 g Mono, 0 g Poly, 7 g Sat); 63 mg Cholesterol; 26 g Carbohydrate; 6 g Fibre; 25 g Protein; 647 mg Sodium*

Arrange eggplant and zucchini on greased baking sheets with sides. Broil on top rack in oven for about 5 minutes per side until browned and softened.

Heat olive oil in large frying pan on medium. Add lamb and turkey. Scramble-fry for about 10 minutes until no longer pink. Drain.

Add next 7 ingredients. Cook for about 10 minutes, stirring often, until carrot is softened. Add tomatoes. Stir. Cook for 5 minutes. Remove from heat.

(continued on next page)

Whisk flour and 1 cup (250 mL) milk in medium saucepan until smooth. Add remaining milk. Cook on medium for about 12 minutes, stirring often, until boiling and thickened. Remove from heat. Stir in feta and Parmesan cheese until melted.

To assemble, layer ingredients in greased 9 x 13 inch (23 x 33 cm) baking dish as follows:

1. 1 cup (250 mL) tomato mixture
2. Eggplant slices, overlapping if necessary
3. Half of remaining tomato mixture
4. Half of cheese mixture
5. Zucchini slices, overlapping if necessary
6. Remaining tomato mixture
7. Remaining cheese mixture

Bake, uncovered, in 350°F (175°C) oven for about 1 hour until bubbling and golden. Let stand for 10 minutes. Cuts into 8 pieces.

Paré Pointer

Good judgment comes from a bad experience—which comes from bad judgment.

Chimichurri Lamb Patties

Lamb is a great nutritional choice because it's high in protein and contains vitamin B12. Chickpeas add nutty flavour and fibre to these South American–style patties.

Canned chickpeas (garbanzo beans), rinsed and drained	1 cup	250 mL
Chopped onion	1 cup	250 mL
Chopped fresh parsley	1/4 cup	60 mL
Chopped fresh cilantro	2 tbsp.	30 mL
Chopped fresh oregano	2 tbsp.	30 mL
Lemon juice	1 tbsp.	15 mL
Garlic cloves, sliced (or 3/4 tsp., 4 mL, powder)	3	3
Dried crushed chilies	1/2 tsp.	2 mL
Salt	1/2 tsp.	2 mL
Pepper	1/4 tsp.	1 mL
Lean ground lamb	3/4 lb.	340 g
Yellow cornmeal	1/2 cup	125 mL

BEFORE: *1 patty:*
554 Calories; **37 g Total Fat** *(15 g Sat); 804 mg Sodium*

AFTER: *1 patty:*
334 Calories; **15 g Total Fat** *(0 g Mono, 0 g Poly, 8 g Sat); 65 mg Cholesterol; 34 g Carbohydrate; 5 g Fibre; 21 g Protein; 488 mg Sodium*

Process first 10 ingredients in food processor with on/off motion until chickpeas are coarsely chopped. Transfer to large bowl.

Add lamb and cornmeal. Mix well. Divide into 4 equal portions. Shape into 4 inch (10 cm) patties. Arrange on greased baking sheet with sides. Broil on top rack in oven for about 4 minutes per side until internal temperature reaches 160°F (71°C). Makes 4 patties.

Mushroom Tarragon Pork

Elegant French flavours of tarragon and Dijon in an easy, nutritious dish.
Try using brown mushrooms for an even prettier look.

Olive (or canola) oil	1 tsp.	5 mL
Pork tenderloin, trimmed of fat and cut into 1/2 inch (12 mm) thick slices	1 lb.	454 g
Sliced fresh white (or brown) mushrooms	2 cups	500 mL
Prepared chicken broth	1 cup	250 mL
Dried tarragon	1 tsp.	5 mL
Pepper	1/8 tsp.	0.5 mL
Cornstarch	1 tbsp.	15 mL
Dijon mustard	1 tbsp.	15 mL
Water	1 tbsp.	15 mL

BEFORE: *1 serving:*
350 Calories; 27 g Total Fat
*(**12 g Sat**); 471 mg Sodium*

AFTER: *1 serving:*
170 Calories; 4 g Total Fat
(2 g Mono, 0 g Poly,
***1 g Sat**);*
65 mg Cholesterol;
5 g Carbohydrate; 0 Fibre;
28 g Protein;
247 mg Sodium

Heat olive oil in large frying pan on medium-high. Add pork. Cook for about 2 minutes per side until browned. Remove to plate. Cover to keep warm.

Add next 4 ingredients to same frying pan. Stir. Bring to a boil, stirring occasionally. Reduce heat to medium. Simmer for about 5 minutes until mushrooms are softened. Add pork.

Combine remaining 3 ingredients in small cup. Add to mushroom mixture. Heat and stir until boiling and thickened. Serves 4.

Apple Sausage Patties

Apple lends subtle tart notes to these moist patties that could be served for brunch or dinner. Cooked patties can be frozen. Reheat from frozen in a 375ºF (190ºC) oven for about 20 minutes until heated through.

Finely chopped celery	1 cup	250 mL
Finely chopped onion	1 cup	250 mL
Grated peeled tart apple (such as Granny Smith)	1 cup	250 mL
Large flake rolled oats	1 cup	250 mL
Dried sage	2 tsp.	10 mL
Fennel seed, crushed	1 tsp.	5 mL
Garlic powder	3/4 tsp.	4 mL
Salt	1 tsp.	5 mL
Pepper	1/2 tsp.	2 mL
Extra-lean ground turkey breast	3/4 lb.	340 g
Lean ground pork	3/4 lb.	340 g
Cooking spray		

Combine first 9 ingredients in large bowl.

Add turkey and pork. Mix well. Using about 1/3 cup (75 mL) for each patty, shape into 1/2 inch (12 mm) thick patties. Arrange on greased baking sheet with sides.

Spray patties with cooking spray. Broil on top rack in oven for about 5 minutes per side until internal temperature reaches 175ºF (80ºC). Makes 14 sausage patties.

BEFORE: *1 sausage patty:* **230 Calories**; *16 g Total Fat (5 g Sat); 301 mg Sodium*

AFTER: *1 sausage patty:* **106 Calories**; *4 g Total Fat (0 g Mono, 0 g Poly, 1.5 g Sat); 27 mg Cholesterol; 7 g Carbohydrate; 1 g Fibre; 10 g Protein; 204 mg Sodium*

Pork Chow Mein

Get your fast-food fix with this full-flavoured, low-fat noodle dish. This chow mein is cooked in the oven with lean pork and plenty of veggies.

Fresh, thin Chinese-style egg noodles	8 oz.	225 g
Boiling water, to cover		
Fresh mixed stir-fry vegetables	6 cups	1.5 L
Boneless centre-cut pork chops, trimmed of fat and cut into thin strips	3/4 lb.	340 g
Prepared vegetable broth	1 1/2 cups	375 mL
Soy sauce	3 tbsp.	50 mL
Cornstarch	2 tbsp.	30 mL
Finely grated ginger root (or 3/4 tsp., 4 mL, ground ginger)	1 tbsp.	15 mL
Garlic cloves, minced (or 1/2 tsp., 2 mL, powder)	2	2
Pepper	1/4 tsp.	1 mL
Fresh bean sprouts	1 cup	250 mL

BEFORE: *1 cup (250 mL): 287 Calories;* **15 g Total Fat** *(4 g Sat); 734 mg Sodium*

AFTER: *1 cup (250 mL): 183 Calories;* **3.5 g Total Fat** *(1 g Mono, 0 g Poly, 1 g Sat); 23 mg Cholesterol; 22 g Carbohydrate; 3 g Fibre; 15 g Protein; 520 mg Sodium*

Place noodles in heatproof large bowl. Pour boiling water over top. Let stand for about 5 minutes until tender. Drain. Cut several times with scissors.

Add vegetables and pork.

Stir next 6 ingredients in small bowl. Pour over noodle mixture. Stir. Transfer to greased 3 quart (3 L) casserole. Bake, covered, in 350°F (175°C) oven for about 40 minutes until vegetables are tender-crisp and sauce is thickened. Stir.

Scatter bean sprouts over top. Stir. Makes about 8 cups (2 L).

Pork Rice Bake

Lots of vegetables, beans and brown rice combine with tender pork in this very attractive casserole. You can use kale or Swiss chard instead of spinach if desired.

Canola oil	2 tsp.	10 mL
Pork tenderloin, trimmed of fat and cut into 1/2 inch (12 mm) pieces	3/4 lb.	340 g
Salt, sprinkle		
Chopped fresh spinach leaves, lightly packed	3 cups	750 mL
Diced butternut squash	2 cups	500 mL
Can of navy beans, rinsed and drained	19 oz.	540 mL
Chopped onion	1 cup	250 mL
Diced celery	1 cup	250 mL
Diced red pepper	1 cup	250 mL
Long-grain brown rice	1 cup	250 mL
Italian seasoning	1 tsp.	5 mL
Pepper	1/4 tsp.	1 mL
Prepared vegetable broth	2 cups	500 mL
Chopped fresh parsley	2 tbsp.	30 mL

BEFORE: *1 cup (250 mL):*
482 Calories; *19 g Total Fat (8.6 g Sat); 2 g Fibre; 956 mg Sodium*

AFTER: *1 cup (250 mL):*
211 Calories; *3 g Total Fat (1 g Mono, 0.5 g Poly, 0 g Sat); 20 mg Cholesterol; 33 g Carbohydrate; 5 g Fibre; 14 g Protein; 250 mg Sodium*

Heat canola oil in large frying pan on medium-high. Add pork. Sprinkle with salt. Cook for about 8 minutes, stirring occasionally, until browned. Transfer to large bowl.

Add next 9 ingredients. Stir. Transfer to greased 9 x 13 inch (23 x 33 cm) baking dish.

Add broth. Cook, covered, in 375°F (190°C) oven for about 1 1/2 hours, stirring at halftime, until rice is tender. Let stand, covered, for 10 minutes.

Sprinkle with parsley. Makes about 9 cups (2.25 L).

Pictured on page 89.

Irish Lentil Stew

A warm, rustic stew that's perfect for those cold, blustery days.

Canola oil	2 tsp.	10 mL
Boneless lamb shoulder, trimmed of fat and cut into 1 inch (2.5 cm) pieces	1 1/2 lbs.	680 g
Garlic powder	1/2 tsp.	2 mL
Pepper	1/4 tsp.	1 mL
Chopped onion	2 cups	500 mL
Dark beer	1 cup	250 mL
Low-sodium prepared chicken broth	3 cups	750 mL
Red baby potatoes, larger ones cut in half	1 1/2 lbs.	680 g
Baby carrots	2 cups	500 mL
Chopped celery	1 1/2 cups	375 mL
Dried green lentils	1 cup	250 mL
Dried thyme	1/2 tsp.	2 mL
Bay leaf	1	1
Chopped fresh parsley	2 tbsp.	30 mL

BEFORE: *1 cup (250 mL):*
393 Calories; 15 g Total Fat (5.1 g Sat); 5 g Fibre;
1056 mg Sodium

AFTER: *1 cup (250 mL):*
290 Calories; 6 g Total Fat (2 g Mono, 0.5 g Poly, 2 g Sat); 54 mg Cholesterol; 35 g Carbohydrate; 6 g Fibre; 23 g Protein;
276 mg Sodium

Heat canola oil in Dutch oven on medium-high. Add lamb. Sprinkle with garlic powder and pepper. Cook for about 10 minutes, stirring occasionally, until browned.

Add onion and beer. Heat and stir for 1 minute, scraping any brown bits from bottom of pot.

Add next 7 ingredients. Stir. Bring to a boil. Reduce heat to medium-low. Simmer, covered, for about 2 hours, stirring occasionally, until lamb is tender. Remove and discard bay leaf.

Sprinkle with parsley. Makes about 9 cups (2.25 L).

Pictured on page 89.

Whiskey Ginger Tenderloin

Choose lean pork tenderloin for your next Sunday night roast.
A dry spice rub gives plenty of flavour.

Ground ginger	2 tsp.	10 mL
Dry mustard	1 tsp.	5 mL
Garlic powder	1 tsp.	5 mL
Salt	1/4 tsp.	1 mL
Pepper	1/4 tsp.	1 mL
Pork tenderloin, trimmed of fat	1 lb.	454 g
Bourbon whiskey	1/4 cup	60 mL
Ginger marmalade	1/4 cup	60 mL

Combine first 5 ingredients in small bowl. Rub over pork. Place on greased foil-lined baking sheet with sides. Cook in 425°F (220°C) oven for about 20 minutes until internal temperature reaches 155°F (68°C).

Combine whiskey and marmalade in microwave-safe small bowl. Microwave on high (100%) for 30 seconds until bubbling (see Tip, page 130). Brush half of mixture over pork. Broil on centre rack in oven for about 5 minutes until starting to brown. Brush with remaining whiskey mixture. Cover with foil. Let stand for 5 minutes. Serves 4.

Pictured on page 125.

BEFORE: *1 serving: 233 Calories; 8.9 Total Fat (2.7 g Sat);* **307 mg Sodium**

AFTER: *1 serving: 237 Calories; 3 g Total Fat (1.5 g Mono, 0 g Poly, 1 g Sat); 67 mg Cholesterol; 15 g Carbohydrate; 0 g Fibre; 28 g Protein;* **210 mg Sodium**

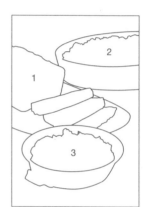

1. Hearty Irish Soda Bread, page 105
2. Pork Rice Bake, page 86
3. Irish Lentil Stew, page 87

Props: Totally Bamboo
Casa Bugatti
Cherison Enterprises

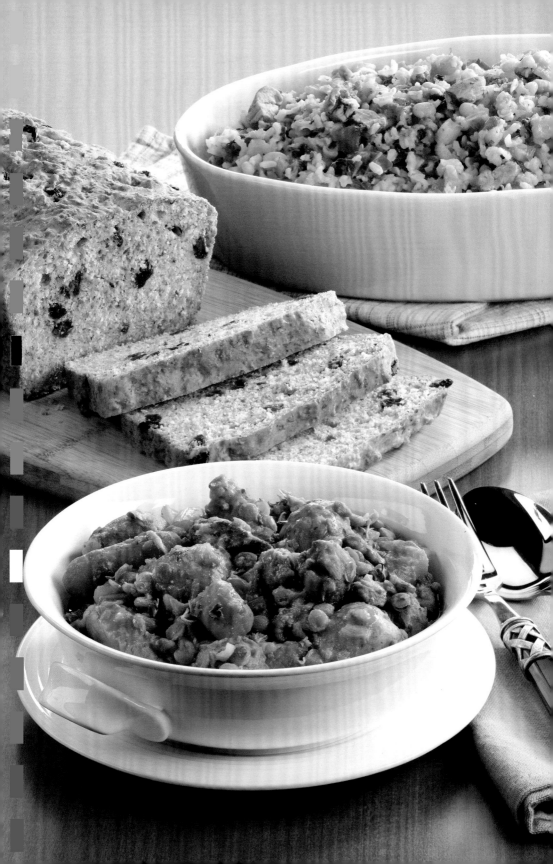

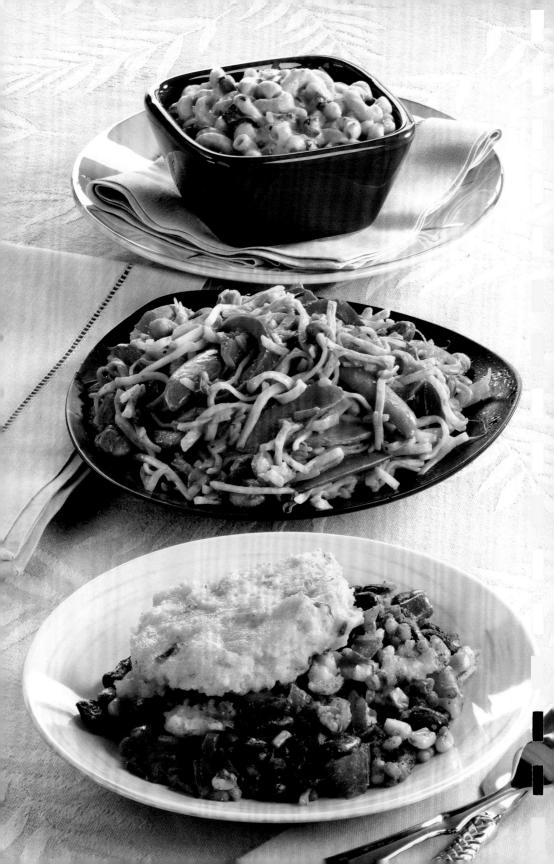

Fettuccine Alfredo

A little butter, milk and reduced-fat cream cheese help to create that creamy,
rich Alfredo sauce that everyone loves—but without all that unhealthy fat.

Water	12 cups	3 L
Salt	1 1/2 tsp.	7 mL
Fettuccine	10 oz.	285 g
Butter	2 tbsp.	30 mL
All-purpose flour	2 tbsp.	30 mL
Milk	1 cup	250 mL
Prepared vegetable broth	1 cup	250 mL
95% fat-free spreadable cream cheese	1/4 cup	60 mL
Coarsely ground pepper	1/2 tsp.	2 mL
Grated Parmesan cheese	3/4 cup	175 mL
Chopped fresh parsley	2 tbsp.	30 mL

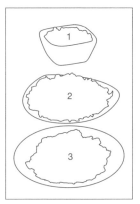

1. Three-Cheese
   Macaroni, page 92
2. Edamame Noodle
   Bowl, page 93
3. Tamale Pie, page 96

Combine water and salt in Dutch oven. Bring to a boil. Add pasta. Boil, uncovered, for 11 to 13 minutes, stirring occasionally, until tender but firm. Drain. Return to same pot. Cover to keep warm.

Melt butter in large saucepan on medium. Add flour. Heat and stir for 1 minute. Slowly add milk, stirring constantly.

Add next 3 ingredients. Cook for about 5 minutes, stirring often, until boiling and slightly thickened. Reduce heat to medium-low. Simmer, uncovered, for 5 minutes, stirring occasionally.

Add Parmesan cheese. Heat and stir until melted. Add pasta. Toss. Transfer to serving bowl.

Sprinkle with parsley. Makes about 5 1/2 cups (1.4 L).

BEFORE: *1 cup (250 mL): 540 Calories; **32 g Total Fat** (19 g Sat); 375 mg Sodium*

AFTER: *1 cup (250 mL): 310 Calories; **8 g Total Fat** (2 g Mono, 0 g Poly, 4.5 g Sat); 23 mg Cholesterol; 43 g Carbohydrate; 1 g Fibre; 13 g Protein; 371 mg Sodium*

Three-Cheese Macaroni

Colourful bits of spinach and red pepper add a touch of fancy flair to this healthy remake of classic macaroni and cheese.

Canola oil	1 tbsp.	15 mL
Finely chopped onion	1 cup	250 mL
Chopped fresh spinach leaves, lightly packed	4 cups	1 L
Finely chopped red pepper	1 cup	250 mL
All-purpose flour	1/4 cup	60 mL
Dry mustard	1/2 tsp.	2 mL
Salt	1/4 tsp.	1 mL
Pepper	1/4 tsp.	1 mL
Skim milk	3 cups	750 mL
Grated sharp Cheddar cheese	2/3 cup	150 mL
Grated Parmesan cheese	1/2 cup	125 mL
Grated Asiago cheese	1/4 cup	60 mL
Water	12 cups	3 L
Salt	1 1/2 tsp.	7 mL
Whole-wheat elbow macaroni	2 1/2 cups	625 mL

BEFORE: *1 cup (250 mL): 470 Calories;* **28 g Total Fat** *(14 g Sat); 896 mg Sodium*

AFTER: *1 cup (250 mL): 280 Calories;* **10 g Total Fat** *(2.5 g Mono, 1 g Poly, 4.5 g Sat); 20 mg Cholesterol; 36 g Carbohydrate; 4 g Fibre; 16 g Protein; 320 mg Sodium*

Heat canola oil in large saucepan on medium. Add onion. Cook for about 5 minutes, stirring often, until softened. Add spinach and red pepper. Cook for about 2 minutes, stirring occasionally, until spinach starts to wilt.

Sprinkle with next 4 ingredients. Heat and stir for 2 minutes. Slowly add milk, stirring constantly. Heat and stir until boiling and thickened. Reduce heat to medium-low.

Add next 3 ingredients. Heat and stir until cheese is melted.

Combine water and salt in Dutch oven. Bring to a boil. Add pasta. Boil, uncovered, for 6 to 8 minutes, stirring occasionally, until tender but firm. Drain. Add to cheese mixture. Stir until coated. Makes about 7 1/2 cups (1.9 L).

Pictured on page 90.

Edamame Noodle Bowl

Thai one on with rice noodles and colourful veggies coated in a smooth, spicy peanut sauce.

Water	8 cups	2 L
Medium rice stick noodles	8 oz.	225 g
Smooth peanut butter	1/2 cup	125 mL
Water	1/2 cup	125 mL
Soy sauce	3 tbsp.	50 mL
Brown sugar, packed	2 tbsp.	30 mL
Lime juice	2 tbsp.	30 mL
Chili paste (sambal oelek)	1/2 tsp.	2 mL
Canola oil	1 tsp.	5 mL
Frozen shelled edamame (soybeans), thawed	2 cups	500 mL
Thinly sliced carrot	1 cup	250 mL
Garlic cloves, minced (or 1/2 tsp., 2 mL, powder)	2	2
Sugar snap peas, trimmed	2 cups	500 mL
Thinly sliced red pepper	1 cup	250 mL
Fresh bean sprouts	2 cups	500 mL

BEFORE: *1 cup (250 mL):*
326 Calories; 10 g Total Fat (12 g Sat); **1339 mg Sodium**

AFTER: *1 cup (250 mL):*
340 Calories; 13 g Total Fat (0 g Mono, 0 g Poly, 2.5 g Sat); 0 mg Cholesterol; 48 g Carbohydrate; 6 g Fibre; 13 g Protein;
546 mg Sodium

Bring water to a boil in large saucepan or Dutch oven. Add noodles. Boil, uncovered, for about 6 minutes, stirring occasionally, until noodles are tender but firm. Drain. Rinse with cold water. Drain well. Return to same pot.

Combine next 6 ingredients in small bowl.

Heat canola oil in large frying pan on medium. Add next 3 ingredients. Cook for about 5 minutes, stirring often, until carrot starts to soften.

Add peas, red pepper and peanut butter mixture. Cook for about 2 minutes, stirring occasionally, until vegetables are tender-crisp.

Add bean sprouts. Cook and stir until heated through. Add to noodles. Toss. Makes about 7 cups (1.75 L).

Pictured on page 90.

Veggie Bean Enchiladas

Hearty lower-fat enchiladas that are packed full of veggies and Mexican flavours, with the perfect amount of tomato and cheese sauce over top.

Canola oil	1 tsp.	5 mL
Chopped fresh brown (or white) mushrooms	2 cups	500 mL
Chopped onion	1 cup	250 mL
Chopped green pepper	1 cup	250 mL
Garlic cloves, minced (or 1/2 tsp., 2 mL, powder)	2	2
Can of black beans, rinsed and drained	19 oz.	540 mL
Frozen kernel corn	1 cup	250 mL
Reserved tomato juice	1/2 cup	125 mL
Red wine vinegar	2 tbsp.	30 mL
Chili powder	1 tbsp.	15 mL
Granulated sugar	1 tsp.	5 mL
Dried crushed chilies	1/2 tsp.	2 mL
Ground cumin	1/2 tsp.	2 mL
Pepper	1/2 tsp.	2 mL
Whole-wheat flour tortillas (10 inch, 25 cm, diameter)	6	6
Can of diced tomatoes, drained and juice reserved	14 oz.	398 mL
Sour cream	2 tbsp.	30 mL
Grated Mexican cheese blend	3/4 cup	175 mL

BEFORE: *1 serving:*
453 Calories; 25.6 g Total Fat (12 g Sat); **3 g Fibre***; 1163 Sodium*

AFTER: *1 serving:*
340 Calories; 13 g Total Fat (6 g Mono, 1.5 g Poly, 4.0 g Sat); 13 mg Cholesterol; 49 g Carbohydrate; **10 g Fibre***; 14 g Protein; 930 mg Sodium*

Heat canola oil in large frying pan on medium. Add next 4 ingredients. Cook for about 10 minutes until onion is softened and mushrooms start to brown.

Mash 1 cup (250 mL) beans in small bowl. Add to mushroom mixture. Add next 8 ingredients and remaining beans. Stir. Cook for about 5 minutes until heated through.

(continued on next page)

Vegetarian

Arrange tortillas on work surface. Spoon about 1/2 cup (125 mL) bean mixture along centre of each tortilla. Roll up tightly from bottom to enclose filling, leaving ends open. Arrange, seam-side down, in greased 9 x 13 inch (23 x 33 cm) baking dish.

Combine tomatoes and sour cream in separate small bowl. Spoon over tortillas. Sprinkle with cheese. Cover with greased foil. Bake in 375°F (190°C) oven for about 40 minutes until heated through. Serves 6.

Pictured on page 72 and on back cover.

Paré Pointer
The best shoes to wear in case of a flood are pumps.

Tamale Pie

Barley is a unique addition to this low-fat, cornmeal-topped remake of Tamale Pie. You can cook a large batch of barley and then freeze it, and then you'll always have some on hand to throw into soups, stews or salads.

Water	8 cups	2 L
Salt	1 tsp.	5 mL
Pot barley	1/3 cup	75 mL
Canola oil	1 tsp.	5 mL
Chopped green pepper	1 cup	250 mL
Chopped onion	1 cup	250 mL
Garlic cloves, minced (or 1/2 tsp., 2 mL, powder)	2	2
Can of kidney beans, rinsed and drained	19 oz.	540 mL
Chopped tomato	1 1/2 cups	375 mL
Frozen kernel corn	1 cup	250 mL
Chili powder	2 tbsp.	30 mL
Dried crushed chilies	1/2 tsp.	2 mL
Salt	1/4 tsp.	1 mL
Water	3 cups	750 mL
Yellow cornmeal	1 cup	250 mL
Grated jalapeño Monterey Jack cheese	1/2 cup	125 mL
Salsa	1/4 cup	60 mL

BEFORE: *1 serving:*
486 Calories; 22 g Total Fat;
4 g Fibre; *843 mg Sodium*

AFTER: *1 serving:*
*288 Calories; 4 g Total Fat
(0.5 g Mono, 0 g Poly,
2 g Sat); 9 mg Cholesterol;
51 g Carbohydrate;*
8 g Fibre; *10 g Protein;
406 mg Sodium*

Combine first amount of water and salt in large saucepan. Bring to a boil. Add barley. Reduce heat to medium. Boil gently, partially covered, for about 35 minutes, stirring occasionally, until tender. Drain.

Heat canola oil in large frying pan on medium. Add next 3 ingredients. Cook for about 5 minutes, stirring occasionally, until onion is softened.

Add next 6 ingredients and barley. Stir. Transfer to ungreased 8 x 8 inch (20 x 20 cm) baking dish.

Bring second amount of water to a boil in medium saucepan. Add cornmeal. Heat and stir for about 5 minutes until mixture thickens and pulls away from side of pan.

(continued on next page)

Vegetarian

Add cheese and salsa. Stir. Pour evenly over barley mixture. Bake in 375°F (190°C) oven for about 35 minutes until heated through and topping is set. Serves 6.

Pictured on page 90.

Potato-Crusted Quiche

Gluten-free and filled with healthy veggies. This elegant and versatile quiche could be a quick and easy supper served with a tossed salad and a glass of wine, or a great brunch dish to start your day.

Olive oil	2 tsp.	10 mL
Diced unpeeled potato	1 1/2 cups	375 mL
Diced red onion	1 cup	250 mL
Diced red pepper	1 cup	250 mL
Diced zucchini (with peel)	1 cup	250 mL
Salt	1/8 tsp.	0.5 mL
Large eggs	4	4
Milk	1 cup	250 mL
Dried oregano	1/4 tsp.	1 mL
Pepper	1/8 tsp.	0.5 mL
Grated sharp Cheddar cheese	1/2 cup	125 mL
Finely chopped tomato	1/2 cup	125 mL
Chopped fresh basil	2 tbsp.	30 mL

BEFORE: *1 wedge:*
***272 Calories**; 19.7 g Total Fat (9.1 g Sat); 387 mg Sodium*

AFTER: *1 wedge:*
***113 Calories**; 5 g Total Fat (2 g Mono, 0.5 g Poly, 2 g Sat); 75 mg Cholesterol; 11 g Carbohydrate; 1 g Fibre; 6 g Protein; 115 mg Sodium*

Heat olive oil in large frying pan on medium. Add potato. Cook, covered, for about 12 minutes, stirring occasionally, until browned and tender. Arrange in single layer in bottom of greased 9 inch (23 cm) deep dish pie plate.

Add next 4 ingredients to same frying pan on medium. Cook for about 5 minutes, stirring occasionally, until onion is softened. Scatter over potato.

Beat next 4 ingredients in small bowl. Pour over vegetables. Sprinkle with cheese. Bake in 375°F (190°C) oven for about 40 minutes until knife inserted in centre of quiche comes out clean. Let stand for 10 minutes.

Sprinkle with tomato and basil. Cuts into 8 wedges.

Vegetable Lasagna

A fantastic low-fat lasagna that's high in fibre and cuts nicely into individual portions. Navy beans provide some extra protein, too.

Olive oil	2 tsp.	10 mL
Sliced fresh white (or brown) mushrooms	3 cups	750 mL
Chopped celery	1 cup	250 mL
Chopped onion	1 cup	250 mL
Garlic cloves, minced (or 1/2 tsp., 2 mL, powder)	2	2
Italian seasoning	1 tsp.	5 mL
Salt	1/2 tsp.	2 mL
Pepper	1/2 tsp.	2 mL
Chopped fresh spinach leaves, lightly packed	6 cups	1.5 L
Cans of navy beans (19 oz., 540 mL, each), rinsed and drained	2	2
Tomato sauce	3 1/2 cups	875 mL
Dry (or alcohol-free) white wine	1/2 cup	125 mL
Water	1/2 cup	125 mL
Granulated sugar	1/2 tsp.	2 mL
Oven-ready whole-grain lasagna noodles	12	12
Grated part-skim mozzarella cheese	1 1/2 cups	375 mL
Grated Parmesan cheese	1/2 cup	125 mL

BEFORE: *1 piece:*
365 Calories; ***22.4 Total Fat*** *(4.3 Sat); 2 g Fibre; 987 mg Sodium*

AFTER: *1 piece:*
256 Calories; ***5 g Total Fat*** *(1.5 g Mono, 0 g Poly, 2.5 g Sat); 9 mg Cholesterol; 38 g Carbohydrate; 7 g Fibre; 14 g Protein; 788 mg Sodium*

Heat olive oil in large frying pan on medium. Add next 7 ingredients. Cook for about 10 minutes, stirring occasionally, until celery is softened.

Add spinach and beans. Stir until spinach is wilted.

Stir next 4 ingredients in medium bowl.

(continued on next page)

To assemble, layer ingredients in greased 9 x 13 inch (23 x 33 cm) baking dish as follows:

1. 1 cup (250 mL) tomato sauce mixture
2. 4 noodles
3. Half of spinach mixture
4. 1 cup (250 mL) tomato sauce mixture
5. 4 noodles
6. Remaining spinach mixture
7. Remaining noodles
8. Remaining tomato sauce mixture

Sprinkle with mozzarella and Parmesan cheese. Cover with greased foil. Bake in 350°F (175°C) oven for 50 minutes until noodles are tender. Remove foil. Bake for about 20 minutes until cheese is golden. Let stand for 10 minutes. Cuts into 12 pieces.

Paré Pointer

Be on the safe side. Pick your friends but not to pieces.

Vegetable Strata

This savoury strata features a great combination of mushrooms, red pepper and zucchini and is lower in fat and sodium. Serve with a tossed green salad.

Canola oil	2 tsp.	10 mL
Sliced fresh brown (or white) mushrooms	2 cups	500 mL
Chopped fennel bulb (white part only)	1 cup	250 mL
Chopped red onion	1 cup	250 mL
Garlic clove, minced (or 1/4 tsp., 1 mL, powder)	1	1
Chopped red pepper	1 cup	250 mL
Diced zucchini (with peel)	1 cup	250 mL
Dried basil	1/2 tsp.	2 mL
Dried oregano	1/2 tsp.	2 mL
Cubed whole-wheat (or multi-grain) baguette, 1 inch (2.5 cm) pieces	6 cups	1.5 L
Grated Italian cheese blend	1 cup	250 mL
Egg whites (large)	4	4
Large eggs	4	4
Milk	2 cups	500 mL
Sun-dried tomato pesto	2 tbsp.	30 mL

BEFORE: *1 serving:*
668 Calories; *46.3 g Total Fat (22 g Sat); 1495 mg Sodium*

AFTER: *1 serving:*
310 Calories; *12 g Total Fat (2 g Mono, 1 g Poly, 3.5 g Sat); 108 mg Cholesterol; 33 g Carbohydrate; 8 g Fibre; 20 g Protein; 490 mg Sodium*

Heat canola oil in large frying pan on medium-high. Add next 4 ingredients. Cook for about 10 minutes, stirring often, until onion is softened and mushrooms start to brown.

Add next 4 ingredients. Cook for about 5 minutes, stirring occasionally, until red pepper is tender-crisp. Transfer to large bowl. Let stand until cool.

Add bread cubes and cheese. Toss. Transfer to greased 9 x 13 inch (23 x 33 cm) baking dish.

Beat remaining 4 ingredients in same large bowl. Pour over bread mixture. Chill, covered, for at least 6 hours or overnight. Bake, uncovered, in 350°F (175°C) oven for about 45 minutes until puffed and golden. Serves 6.

Eggplant Parmigiana

This slimmed-down version is already much lower in fat and sodium than the traditional version with breaded, fried eggplant. You can reduce the fat even more by choosing a reduced-fat cheese. Serve with a leafy green salad and crusty bread.

Can of diced tomatoes (with juice)	28 oz.	796 mL
Dry (or alcohol-free) white wine	1/4 cup	60 mL
Tomato paste (see Tip, page 32)	3 tbsp.	50 mL
Dried basil	1 1/2 tsp.	7 mL
Dried oregano	1 1/2 tsp.	7 mL
Garlic cloves, minced (or 1/2 tsp., 2 mL, powder)	2	2
Medium eggplants (with peel), about 1 1/4 lbs. (560 g) each	2	2
Salt, sprinkle		
Pepper, sprinkle		
Grated Italian cheese blend	1 1/3 cups	325 mL
Grated Parmesan cheese	1/4 cup	60 mL

BEFORE: *1 piece:*
*291 Calories; 18 g Total Fat
(5 g Sat);* **1379 mg Sodium**

AFTER: *1 piece:*
*160 Calories; 6 g Total Fat
(0 g Mono, 0 g Poly,
3.5 g Sat);
18 mg Cholesterol;
19 g Carbohydrate;
7 g Fibre; 10 g Protein;*
679 mg Sodium

Process first 6 ingredients in blender or food processor until smooth.

Slice eggplants crosswise, about 1/4 inch (6 mm) thick. Discard outer slices. Arrange in single layer on greased baking sheets with sides. Sprinkle both sides with salt and pepper. Broil on centre rack in oven for about 8 minutes per side until browned and softened.

To assemble, layer ingredients in greased 9 x 13 inch (23 x 33 cm) baking dish as follows:

1. 1/3 of tomato mixture
2. Half of eggplant slices, overlapping if necessary
3. Half of Italian cheese blend
4. 1/3 of tomato mixture
5. Remaining eggplant slices, overlapping if necessary
6. Remaining tomato mixture
7. Remaining Italian cheese blend

Sprinkle with Parmesan cheese. Bake, uncovered, in 350°F (175°C) oven for about 45 minutes until cheese is golden. Let stand for 10 minutes. Cuts into 6 pieces.

Vegetarian

Veggieloaf Muffins

Try going meatless at least once a week for a healthier diet. And try these wholesome veggie "muffins" as a main or a side—they're hearty, flavourful and reminiscent of meatloaf.

Prepared vegetable broth	3/4 cup	175 mL
Quinoa, rinsed avnd drained	1/2 cup	125 mL
Canola oil	2 tsp.	10 mL
Finely chopped portobello mushrooms	2 cups	500 mL
Finely chopped onion	1 cup	250 mL
Grated zucchini (with peel)	3/4 cup	175 mL
Chopped fresh oregano	1 tsp.	5 mL
(or 1/4 tsp., 1 mL, dried)		
Montreal steak spice	1/2 tsp.	2 mL
Garlic clove, minced	1	1
(or 1/4 tsp., 1 mL, powder)		
Dried crushed chilies	1/4 tsp.	1 mL
Salt	1/4 tsp.	1 mL
Can of lentils, rinsed and drained	19 oz.	540 mL
Tomato paste (see Tip, page 32)	2 tbsp.	30 mL
Balsamic vinegar	1 tbsp.	15 mL
Large eggs, fork-beaten	2	2
Quick-cooking rolled oats	3/4 cup	175 mL

BEFORE: *1 muffin:*
*446 Calories; 31 g Total Fat (**12 g Sat**); 977 mg Sodium*

AFTER: *1 muffin:*
*117 Calories; 2.5 g Total Fat (0.9 g Mono, 0.5 g Poly, **0.4 g Sat**); 35 mg Cholesterol; 18 g Carbohydrate; 5 g Fibre; 6 g Protein; 171 mg Sodium*

Bring broth to a boil in small saucepan. Add quinoa. Stir. Reduce heat to medium-low. Simmer, covered, for about 20 minutes, without stirring, until quinoa is tender and liquid is absorbed. Transfer to large bowl.

Heat canola oil in large frying pan on medium. Add mushrooms and onion. Cook for about 8 minutes, stirring often, until onion starts to soften.

Add next 6 ingredients. Heat and stir for about 1 minute until garlic is fragrant. Add to quinoa. Stir.

Mash lentils in medium bowl. Add tomato paste and vinegar. Stir well. Add to quinoa mixture.

(continued on next page)

Add eggs and rolled oats. Mix well. Fill 12 greased muffin cups 1/2 full. Cook in 350°F (175°C) oven for about 20 minutes until browned and internal temperature reaches 165°F (74°C). Run knife around inside edge of muffin cups to loosen. Makes 12 muffins.

Pepper Quinoa Pizza

Instead of a high-fat, high-sodium normal pizza crust, try this distinctive and delicious quinoa crust that is protein-packed and gluten-free!

Prepared vegetable broth	1 3/4 cups	425 mL
Quinoa, rinsed and drained	1 1/4 cups	300 mL
Cornstarch	1/4 cup	60 mL
Basil pesto	2 tbsp.	30 mL
Canola oil	2 tbsp.	30 mL
Yellow cornmeal	2 tbsp.	30 mL
Tomato sauce	1/2 cup	125 mL
Thinly sliced fresh white mushrooms	1 cup	250 mL
Diced red pepper	1 cup	250 mL
Diced yellow pepper	1/2 cup	125 mL
Grated Asiago cheese	3/4 cup	175 mL

BEFORE: *1 wedge:*
380 Calories, **23 g Total Fat** *(8 g Sat);*
930 mg Sodium

AFTER: *1 wedge:*
230 Calories; **12 g Total Fat** *(2 g Mono, 1 g Poly, 3.5 g Sat);*
15 mg Cholesterol;
24 g Carbohydrate;
2 g Fibre; 7 g Protein;
410 mg Sodium

Bring broth to a boil in medium saucepan. Add quinoa. Stir. Reduce heat to medium-low. Simmer, covered, for about 20 minutes, without stirring, until quinoa is tender and liquid is absorbed. Spread on large plate. Let stand until cool. Transfer to food processor.

Add next 3 ingredients. Process until combined and mixture resembles dough.

Sprinkle cornmeal over well-greased 12 inch (30 cm) pizza pan. Press quinoa mixture into pan. Bake on bottom rack in 450°F (230°C) oven for about 15 minutes until set and edges are dry.

Spread tomato sauce over crust. Scatter remaining 4 ingredients, in order given, over tomato sauce. Bake for about 20 minutes until cheese is melted and golden. Cuts into 8 wedges.

Pictured on page 107.

Nutty Cheese Patties

These perfectly seasoned patties are filled with two grains, Cheddar cheese and lots of veggies. Serve on multi-grain or whole-wheat buns with your favourite burger toppings, or on their own with a leafy green salad.

Canola oil	1 tsp.	5 mL
Chopped celery	1 cup	250 mL
Chopped fresh brown (or white) mushrooms	1 cup	250 mL
Chopped onion	1 cup	250 mL
Grated carrot	1 cup	250 mL
Garlic cloves, minced (or 1/2 tsp., 2 mL, powder	2	2
Prepared vegetable broth	1 cup	250 mL
Bulgur	1/2 cup	125 mL
Salt	1/2 tsp.	2 mL
Pepper	1/4 tsp.	1 mL
Cooked brown rice (about 2/3 cup, 150 mL, uncooked)	2 cups	500 mL
Chopped pecans, toasted (see Tip, page 110)	1 cup	250 mL
Chopped fresh parsley (or 1 tbsp., 15 mL, flakes)	1/4 cup	60 mL
Grated sharp Cheddar cheese	1 cup	250 mL
Yellow cornmeal	1/2 cup	125 mL

BEFORE: *1 patty:*
448 Calories; 24.8 g Total Fat (12 g Sat); 1470 mg Sodium

AFTER: *1 patty:*
267 Calories; 14 g Total Fat (7 g Mono, 3 g Poly, 3.5 g Sat); 15 mg Cholesterol; 29 g Carbohydrate; 5 g Fibre; 8 g Protein; 297 mg Sodium

Heat canola oil in large frying pan on medium. Add next 5 ingredients. Cook for about 10 minutes, stirring occasionally, until celery is softened.

Add broth. Bring to a boil. Add next 3 ingredients. Stir. Reduce heat to medium-low. Cook, covered, for about 20 minutes until bulgur is tender and liquid is absorbed. Transfer half of bulgur mixture to food processor.

Add half of rice. Add pecans and parsley. Process with on/off motion until mixture is coarsely chopped and combined. Transfer to large bowl.

Add cheese, cornmeal, remaining bulgur mixture and remaining rice. Stir. Using about 1/2 cup (125 mL) for each, shape into 4 inch (10 cm) patties. Arrange on greased baking sheets with sides. Bake in 350°F (175°C) oven for about 15 minutes per side until browned. Makes about 9 patties.

Vegetarian

Hearty Irish Soda Bread

A rustic, golden, better-for-you loaf full of sweet raisins. Perfect served up for breakfast with jam, or served with lunch to accompany a bowl of soup.

All-purpose flour	1 1/2 cups	375 mL
Whole-wheat flour	1 1/2 cups	375 mL
Dark raisins	1/2 cup	125 mL
Wheat germ, toasted (see Tip, below)	1/4 cup	60 mL
Brown sugar, packed	2 tbsp.	30 mL
Baking soda	1 1/2 tsp.	7 mL
Caraway seed	1 tsp.	5 mL
Salt	3/4 tsp.	4 mL
1% buttermilk (or soured milk, see Tip, page 136)	1 1/2 cups	375 mL
Low-fat plain yogurt	1/2 cup	125 mL
Canola oil	1/4 cup	60 mL

BEFORE: *1 slice:*
160 Calories; 7 g Total Fat
*(**4 g Sat**); 331 mg Sodium*

AFTER: *1 slice:*
157 Calories; 4 g Total Fat
(2 g Mono, 1 g Poly,
***0 g Sat**); 3 mg Cholesterol;*
25 g Carbohydrate;
2 g Fibre; 4 g Protein;
255 mg Sodium

Combine first 8 ingredients in large bowl. Make a well in centre.

Combine remaining 3 ingredients in small bowl. Add to well. Stir until just moistened. Spread evenly in greased 9 x 5 x 3 inch (22 x 12.5 x 7.5 cm) loaf pan. Bake in 350°F (175°C) oven for about 50 minutes until wooden pick inserted in centre comes out clean. Let stand in pan for 10 minutes before removing to wire rack to cool. Cuts into 16 slices.

Pictured on page 89.

 To toast wheat germ, spread evenly in an ungreased shallow frying pan. Heat and stir on medium until golden. To bake, spread evenly in an ungreased shallow pan. Bake in a 350°F (175°C) oven for 3 minutes, stirring or shaking often, until golden. Cool before adding to recipe.

Wild Rice Butternut Latkes

This makeover of potato pancakes adds creamy butternut squash and textured wild rice. Serve with roast pork, chicken or salmon.

Water	6 cups	1.5 L
Salt	1/4 tsp.	1 mL
Wild rice	1/3 cup	75 mL
Grated butternut squash, squeezed dry	1 1/2 cups	375 mL
Grated peeled potato, squeezed dry	1 cup	250 mL
All-purpose flour	1/4 cup	60 mL
Thinly sliced green onion	1/4 cup	60 mL
Large egg, fork-beaten	1	1
Dried sage	1/4 tsp.	1 mL
Salt	1/4 tsp.	1 mL
Pepper	1/8 tsp.	0.5 mL
Canola oil	1/4 cup	60 mL

Combine water and salt in medium saucepan. Bring to a boil. Add wild rice. Stir. Reduce heat to medium. Boil gently, partially covered, for about 35 minutes until rice is tender. Drain.

Combine next 8 ingredients in large bowl. Add rice. Stir well.

Heat 2 tbsp. (30 mL) canola oil in large frying pan on medium. Drop 5 portions of potato mixture into pan, using 1/4 cup (60 mL) for each. Press down lightly to 3 inch (7.5 cm) rounds. Cook for about 3 minutes per side until browned. Transfer to paper towel-lined plate to drain. Cover to keep warm. Repeat with remaining canola oil and rice mixture. Makes about 10 latkes.

Pictured on page 108.

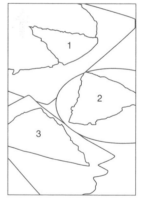

1. Tuna Melt Pizza, page 77
2. Pepper Quinoa Pizza, page 103
3. Beefy Mushroom Pizza, page 46

Props: Totally Bamboo

BEFORE: *1 latke: 181 Calories; **12 g Total Fat** (1 g Sat); 157 mg Sodium*

AFTER: *1 latke: 105 Calories; **6 g Total Fat** (3.5 g Mono, 1.5 g Poly, 0.5 g Sat); 14 mg Cholesterol; 12 g Carbohydrate; 1 g Fibre; 2 g Protein; 65 mg Sodium*

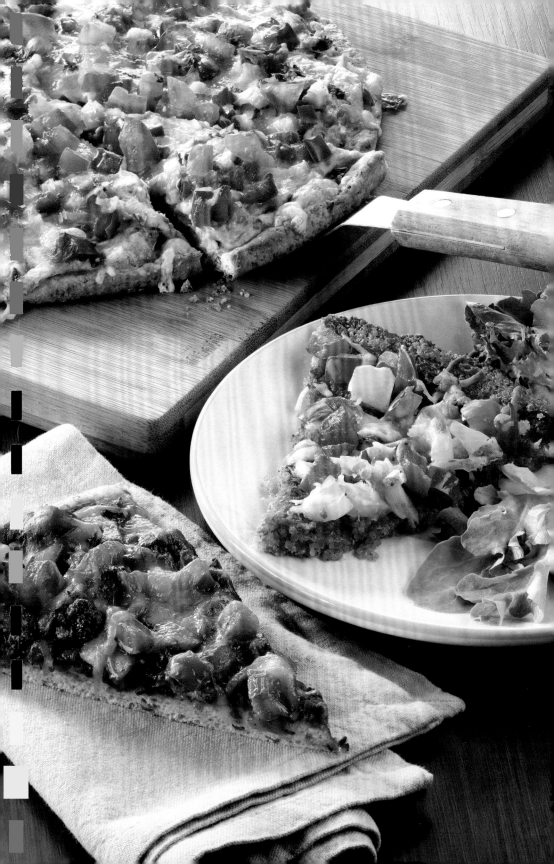

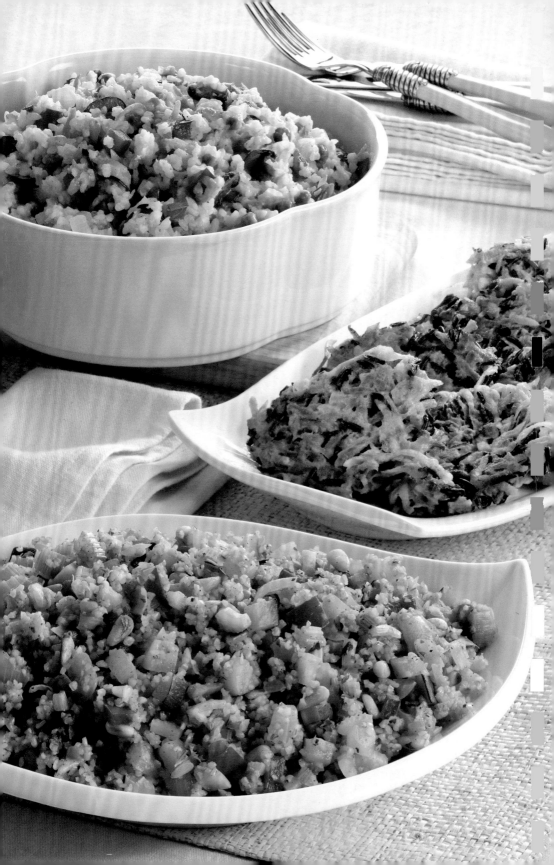

Garden Risotto

A traditional-looking risotto that's baked in the oven instead of on the stove,
so there's no need to add oil. Sure to impress your guests.

Arborio rice	1 cup	250 mL
Chopped onion	1 cup	250 mL
Diced red pepper	1 cup	250 mL
Grated carrot	1 cup	250 mL
Thinly sliced fresh brown (or white) mushrooms	1 cup	250 mL
Pepper	1/4 tsp.	1 mL
Prepared vegetable broth, hot	2 3/4 cup	675 mL
Frozen peas, thawed	1 cup	250 mL
Grated Parmesan cheese	1/4 cup	60 mL
Chopped fresh parsley (or 3/4 tsp., 4 mL, flakes)	1 tbsp.	15 mL
White wine vinegar	2 tsp.	10 mL

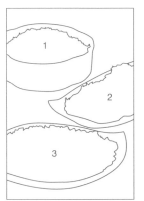

Combine first 6 ingredients in greased 2 quart (2 L) casserole. Add broth. Stir. Cook, covered, in 400°F (205°C) oven for about 35 minutes, stirring at halftime, until rice is tender.

Add remaining 4 ingredients. Stir. Let stand, covered, for 5 minutes. Makes about 6 cups (1.5 L).

Pictured at left.

1. Garden Risotto, above
2. Wild Rice Butternut Latkes, page 106
3. Herb Bulgur Pilaf, page 110

Props: Cherison Enterprises
Moderno
Casa Bugatti

BEFORE: *1/2 cup (125 mL):* **193 Calories***; 6 g Total Fat (3 g Sat); 528 mg Sodium*

AFTER: *1/2 cup (125 mL):* **89 Calories***; 1 g Total Fat (0 g Mono, 0 g Poly, 0 g Sat); 0 mg Cholesterol; 18 g Carbohydrate; 1 g Fibre; 3 g Protein; 170 mg Sodium*

Herb Bulgur Pilaf

Mediterranean-style flavours in a colourful pilaf topped with pine nuts and parsley. Bulgur is quick and easy to cook, and also low in fat and high in calcium.

Canola oil	1 tsp.	5 mL
Chopped onion	1 cup	250 mL
Diced celery	1 cup	250 mL
Garlic cloves, minced (or 1/2 tsp., 2 mL, powder)	2	2
Diced zucchini (with peel)	1 cup	250 mL
Diced red pepper	1/2 cup	125 mL
Prepared vegetable broth	1 1/2 cups	375 mL
Italian seasoning	1 tsp.	5 mL
Pepper	1/4 tsp.	1 mL
Bulgur	3/4 cup	175 mL
Pine nuts, toasted (see Tip, below)	1 tbsp.	15 mL
Chopped fresh parsley	1 tbsp.	15 mL

BEFORE: *1/2 cup (125 mL):*
141 Calories; 5 g Total Fat (2 g Sat); 1 g Fibre;
516 mg Sodium

AFTER: *1/2 cup (125 mL):*
110 Calories; 2 g Total Fat (1 g Mono, 1 g Poly, 0 g Sat); 0 mg Cholesterol; 21 g Carbohydrate; 3 g Fibre; 4 g Protein;
168 mg Sodium

Heat canola oil in large frying pan on medium. Add next 3 ingredients. Cook for about 8 minutes, stirring occasionally, until celery is softened.

Add zucchini and red pepper. Cook for about 5 minutes, stirring occasionally, until red pepper is tender-crisp.

Add next 3 ingredients. Bring to a boil. Add bulgur. Stir. Cook, covered, for about 10 minutes until bulgur is tender and liquid is absorbed.

Sprinkle with pine nuts and parsley. Makes about 3 cups (750 mL).

Pictured on page 108.

 tip When toasting nuts, seeds, oats or coconut, cooking times will vary for each type—so never toast them together. For small amounts, place ingredient in an ungreased shallow frying pan. Heat on medium for 3 to 5 minutes, stirring often, until golden. For larger amounts, spread ingredient evenly in an ungreased shallow pan. Bake in a 350°F (175°C) oven for 5 to 10 minutes, stirring or shaking often, until golden.

Sausage Fruit Stuffing

Italian sausage adds the perfect amount of seasoning to this low-fat stuffing update. You can use apple juice or more chicken broth in place of wine if you prefer.

Multi-grain (or whole-wheat) bread cubes	5 cups	1.25 L
Hot Italian sausage, casing removed	4 oz.	113 g
Chopped onion	1 1/2 cups	375 mL
Diced celery	1 cup	250 mL
Diced unpeeled tart apple (such as Granny Smith)	1 1/2 cups	375 mL
Finely chopped dried figs	1/2 cup	125 mL
Dried thyme	1 tsp.	5 mL
Dried rosemary, crushed	1/2 tsp.	2 mL
Dried sage	1/2 tsp.	2 mL
Prepared chicken broth	1 cup	250 mL
Dry (or alcohol-free) white wine	1/2 cup	125 mL

BEFORE: *1 cup (250 mL): 397 Calories; 21 g Total Fat (7 g Sat);* **2 g Fibre***; 1109 mg Sodium*

AFTER: *1 cup (250 mL): 240 Calories; 6 g Total Fat (0 g Mono, 0 g Poly, 2 g Sat); 10 mg Cholesterol; 36 g Carbohydrate;* **8 g Fibre***; 9 g Protein; 430 mg Sodium*

Arrange bread cubes in single layer on ungreased baking sheet with sides. Bake in 325°F (160°C) oven for about 15 minutes until edges are dry. Transfer to large bowl.

Heat large frying pan on medium. Add next 3 ingredients. Scramble-fry for about 12 minutes until sausage is browned.

Add next 5 ingredients. Heat and stir for 1 minute. Add to bread. Stir.

Drizzle with broth and wine. Stir until moistened. Transfer to greased shallow 2 quart (2 L) casserole. Bake, covered, for 20 minutes. Remove cover. Bake for about 20 minutes until browned. Makes about 7 cups (1.75 L).

Artichoke Potato Peppers

Instead of stuffed potatoes, try stuffed red peppers with a potato, artichoke and bean purée filling. Lots of fibre and flavour.

Chopped peeled potato	2 cups	500 mL
Chopped onion	1/2 cup	125 mL
Garlic clove, minced (or 1/4 tsp., 1 mL, powder)	1	1
Canned white kidney beans, rinsed and drained	1 cup	250 mL
Chopped fresh parsley	2 tbsp.	30 mL
Lemon juice	1 tbsp.	15 mL
Olive (or canola) oil	1 tbsp.	15 mL
Grated lemon zest (see Tip, page 151)	1/2 tsp.	2 mL
Salt	1/4 tsp.	1 mL
Pepper	1/4 tsp.	1 mL
Coarsely chopped marinated artichoke hearts	1/2 cup	125 mL
Small red peppers, halved lengthwise	3	3
Olive oil	1 tsp.	5 mL

BEFORE: *1 stuffed pepper half:* 339 Calories; 18 g Total Fat (**9 g Sat**); 734 mg Sodium

AFTER: *1 stuffed pepper half:* 125 Calories; 3 g Total Fat (2 g Mono, 0 g Poly, **0 g Sat**); 0 mg Cholesterol; 21 g Carbohydrate; 5 g Fibre; 4 g Protein; 207 mg Sodium

Pour water into large saucepan until 1 inch (2.5 cm) deep. Add first 3 ingredients. Cover. Bring to a boil. Boil gently for 12 to 15 minutes until tender. Drain. Transfer potato mixture to food processor.

Add next 7 ingredients. Carefully process until smooth (see Safety Tip). Add artichokes. Process until almost smooth.

Fill pepper halves. Place on ungreased baking sheet with sides. Brush with second amount of olive oil. Bake in 425°F (220°C) oven for about 30 minutes until filling is heated through and peppers are tender-crisp. Makes 6 stuffed pepper halves.

Safety Tip: Follow manufacturer's instructions for processing hot liquids.

Spiced Corn Cakes

Serve this all-purpose side whenever you'd normally serve biscuits, hash browns or potato cakes. Use gluten-free baking powder to make these corn cakes gluten-free.

Yellow cornmeal	2 cups	500 mL
Chopped fresh cilantro (or parsley)	2 tbsp.	30 mL
Chili powder	1 tbsp.	15 mL
Granulated sugar	1 tbsp.	15 mL
Baking soda	1 tsp.	5 mL
Dried crushed chilies (optional)	1/2 tsp.	2 mL
Salt	1/2 tsp.	2 mL
Canned navy beans, rinsed and drained	1 cup	250 mL
Large eggs	2	2
Lime juice	1/4 cup	60 mL
Canola oil	2 tbsp.	30 mL
Fresh (or frozen, thawed) kernel corn	1 cup	250 mL
Chopped red onion	1/2 cup	125 mL
Chopped red pepper	1/2 cup	125 mL
Canola oil	1 tbsp.	30 mL

BEFORE: *1 cake:*
*200 Calories; **9 g Total Fat** (3.5 g Sat); 400 mg Sodium*

AFTER: *1 cake:*
*156 Calories; **4 g Total Fat** (2 g Mono, 1 g Poly, 0 g Sat); 20 mg Cholesterol; 26 g Carbohydrate; 2 g Fibre; 4 g Protein; 221 mg Sodium*

Combine first 7 ingredients in large bowl. Make a well in centre.

Process next 4 ingredients in blender or food processor until smooth.

Add next 3 ingredients. Process until coarsely chopped. Add to well. Stir until combined.

Preheat griddle to medium-high (see Note). Heat 1 1/2 tsp. (7 mL) canola oil on griddle until hot. Drop batter onto griddle, using about 1/4 cup (60 mL) for each cake. Flatten into 3 inch (7.5 cm) diameter patties. Cook for about 3 minutes per side until browned. Transfer to plate. Cover to keep warm. Repeat with remaining batter, heating remaining canola oil on griddle to prevent sticking. Makes about 14 cakes.

Note: If you don't have an electric griddle, use a large frying pan. Heat 1 tsp. (5 mL) canola oil on medium. Heat more canola oil with each batch if necessary to prevent sticking.

Vegetable Fried Rice

Edamame and sesame seeds add a fresh twist to this fried rice dish that's almost like a stir-fry. Great orangey flavour.

Canola oil	1 tbsp.	15 mL
Chopped onion	1/2 cup	125 mL
Diced celery	1/2 cup	125 mL
Grated carrot	1/2 cup	125 mL
Finely grated ginger root (or 1/2 tsp., 2 mL, ground ginger)	2 tsp.	10 mL
Garlic clove, minced (or 1/4 tsp., 1 mL, powder)	1	1
Cooked long-grain brown rice (about 2/3 cup, 150 mL, uncooked)	2 cups	500 mL
Frozen shelled edamame (soybeans), thawed	1 cup	250 mL
Chopped red pepper	1/2 cup	125 mL
Frozen concentrated orange juice, thawed	3 tbsp.	50 mL
Soy sauce	1 tbsp.	15 mL
Rice vinegar	2 tsp.	10 mL
Chili paste (sambal oelek)	1 tsp.	5 mL
Sesame oil (for flavour)	1 tsp.	5 mL
Sliced green onion	2 tbsp.	30 mL
Roasted sesame seeds	1 tbsp.	15 mL

BEFORE: *1/2 cup (125 mL): 203 Calories; 6.8 g Total Fat;* **478 mg Sodium**

AFTER: *1/2 cup (125 mL): 130 Calories; 4 g Total Fat (1.5 g Mono, 1 g Poly, 0 g Sat); 0 mg Cholesterol; 20 g Carbohydrate; 2 g Fibre; 4 g Protein;* **147 mg Sodium**

Heat canola oil in large frying pan on medium. Add next 5 ingredients. Cook for about 10 minutes, stirring often, until celery is softened.

Add next 3 ingredients. Cook for about 5 minutes, stirring often, until red pepper is tender-crisp.

Combine next 5 ingredients in small bowl. Add to rice mixture. Stir. Cook for about 1 minute until heated through. Transfer to serving bowl.

Sprinkle with green onion and sesame seeds. Makes about 4 cups (1 L).

Triple-Chili Oven Fries

Baked instead of deep-fried for a guilt-free and delicious way to enjoy French fries! Try all of the variations and see which seasoning tickles your fancy.

Medium unpeeled yellow potatoes (such as Yukon Gold)	3	3
CHILI SPICE MIX		
Canola oil	1 tbsp.	15 mL
Chili powder	1 tsp.	5 mL
Chili paste (sambal oelek)	1/2 tsp.	2 mL
Dried crushed chilies	1/2 tsp.	2 mL
Salt	1/4 tsp.	1 mL

BEFORE: *1/2 cup (125 mL):* ***310 Calories****; 12 g Total Fat (3 g Sat); 460 mg Sodium*

AFTER: *1/2 cup (125 mL):* ***90 Calories****; 2 g Total Fat (1.5 g Mono, 0.5 g Poly, 0 g Sat); 0 mg Cholesterol; 17 g Carbohydrate; 2 g Fibre; 2 g Protein; 117 mg Sodium*

Cut potatoes lengthwise into 1/2 inch (12 mm) thick slices. Cut slices lengthwise into 1/2 inch (12 mm) thick pieces to make fries.

Chili Spice Mix: Combine all 5 ingredients in large bowl. Add potatoes. Toss to coat. Spread in single layer on ungreased baking sheet with sides. Bake in 450°F (230°C) oven for about 25 minutes, turning once, until crisp and tender. Makes about 3 cups (750 mL).

BARBECUE OVEN FRIES: For the spice mix, omit chili paste and dried crushed chilies. Add 1/2 tsp. (2 mL) packed brown sugar, 1/2 tsp. (2 mL) celery seed, 1/2 tsp. (2 mL) garlic powder, 1/2 tsp. (2 mL) paprika and 1/4 tsp. (1 mL) pepper. Increase salt to 1/2 tsp (2 mL).

HERB GARLIC OVEN FRIES: For the spice mix, omit chili powder and dried crushed chilies. Add 2 tsp. (10 mL) Italian seasoning and 1 tsp. (5 mL) garlic powder.

CURRY OVEN FRIES: For the spice mix, omit chili powder and dried crushed chilies. Add 1 tsp. (5 mL) hot curry powder and 1/2 tsp. (2 mL) packed brown sugar.

Sweet Potato Casserole

Traditional sweet potato casserole gets a modern, healthier overhaul. Sweet potato is spiced up with tropical flavours and topped with toasted oats and pumpkin seeds. Serve with chicken, pork or grilled seafood.

Canola oil	1 tbsp.	15 mL
Chili paste (sambal oelek)	1 tsp.	5 mL
Garlic cloves, minced (or 1/2 tsp., 2 mL, powder)	2	2
Brown sugar, packed	1 tbsp.	15 mL
Finely grated ginger root (or 1/2 tsp., 2 mL, ground ginger)	2 tsp.	10 mL
Dried thyme	1/2 tsp.	2 mL
Ground allspice	1/2 tsp.	2 mL
Ground cinnamon	1/4 tsp.	1 mL
Salt	1/2 tsp.	2 mL
Pepper	1/4 tsp.	1 mL
Cubed peeled orange-fleshed sweet potato	6 cups	1.5 L
Quick-cooking rolled oats, toasted (see Tip, page 110)	1/2 cup	125 mL
Chopped unsalted toasted pumpkin seeds (see Tip, page 110)	1/4 cup	60 mL
Medium unsweetened coconut	2 tbsp.	30 mL
Butter, melted	2 tbsp.	30 mL

BEFORE: *1/2 cup (125 mL):*
352 Calories; *17.9 Total Fat (8.1 g Sat); 360 mg Sodium*

AFTER: *1/2 cup (125 mL):*
146 Calories; *5 g Total Fat (1.5 g Mono, 1 g Poly, 2.5 g Sat);*
5 mg Cholesterol;
23 g Carbohydrate;
3 g Fibre; 2 g Protein;
191 mg Sodium

Combine first 10 ingredients in large bowl.

Add sweet potato. Stir to coat. Transfer to greased 2 quart (2 L) casserole. Bake, covered, in 375°F (190°C) oven for about 40 minutes until sweet potato is tender.

Combine remaining 4 ingredients in small bowl. Spoon over sweet potato mixture. Bake, uncovered, for about 15 minutes until topping is crisp and golden. Makes about 5 cups (1.25 L).

Roasted Cauliflower Mash

A fresh change from boring old mashed potatoes. Garlic adds a deep, layered flavour to potato and cauliflower.

Canola oil	1 tbsp.	15 mL
Cauliflower florets	4 cups	1 L
Garlic cloves, halved	3	3
Chopped peeled potato	4 cups	1 L
1% buttermilk	1/3 cup	75 mL
Salt	1/4 tsp.	1 mL
White (or black) pepper	1/4 tsp.	1 mL

BEFORE: *1/2 cup (125 mL):*
168 Calories; **8 g Total Fat**
(5 g Sat); 328 mg Sodium

AFTER: *1/2 cup (125 mL):*
90 Calories; **1.5 g Total Fat** *(1 g Mono, 0 g Poly, 0 g Sat); 0 mg Cholesterol; 17 g Carbohydrate; 2 g Fibre; 3 g Protein; 92 mg Sodium*

Toss first 3 ingredients in large bowl. Spread on ungreased baking sheet with sides. Cook in 425°F (220°C) oven for about 20 minutes, stirring at halftime, until tender. Transfer to food processor. Process until finely chopped.

Pour water into large saucepan until about 1 inch (2.5 cm) deep. Add potato. Cover. Bring to a boil. Reduce heat to medium. Boil gently for 12 to 15 minutes until tender. Add to cauliflower mixture.

Add remaining 3 ingredients. Carefully process until smooth and creamy (see Safety Tip). Makes about 4 1/2 cups (1.1 L).

Safety Tip: Follow manufacturer's instructions for processing hot liquids.

Broccoflower Bake

Bright green broccoli and tender cauliflower in a creamy low-fat herb sauce that's topped with golden cheese crumbs. An appetizing presentation and a rich taste.

Water	10 cups	2.5 L
Broccoli florets	3 cups	750 mL
Cauliflower florets	3 cups	750 mL
Prepared vegetable broth	1/4 cup	60 mL
All-purpose flour	2 tbsp.	30 mL
Can of 2% evaporated milk	13 1/2 oz.	385 mL
Italian seasoning	1 tsp.	5 mL
Pepper	1/4 tsp.	1 mL
Fresh whole-wheat bread crumbs	1/2 cup	125 mL
Grated Parmesan cheese	1/3 cup	75 mL
Grated Asiago cheese	1/4 cup	60 mL
Canola oil	1 tbsp.	15 mL

BEFORE: *1 serving:*
231 Calories; 16 g Total Fat
(9 g Sat); 499 mg Sodium

AFTER: *1 serving:*
160 Calories; 6 g Total Fat
(1.5 g Mono, 1 g Poly,
2 g Sat); 4 mg Cholesterol;
19 g Carbohydrate;
2 g Fibre; 10 g Protein;
207 mg Sodium

Bring water to a boil in Dutch oven. Add broccoli and cauliflower. Boil for about 3 minutes until tender-crisp. Drain well. Transfer to greased shallow 2 quart (2 L) casserole.

Whisk broth and flour in small saucepan until smooth. Whisk in milk. Add seasoning and pepper. Cook on medium, stirring occasionally, until boiling and thickened. Pour over vegetables.

Combine remaining 4 ingredients in small bowl. Sprinkle over vegetable mixture. Bake, uncovered, in 400°F (205°C) oven for about 25 minutes until bubbling and topping is golden. Serves 6.

Pictured on page 125.

Smoky Cheese Potato Scallop

Another satisfying favourite that's now low in fat and calories. Smoked Gouda cheese adds a distinct flavour and really makes this one memorable.

Prepared chicken broth	1/2 cup	125 mL
All-purpose flour	2 tbsp.	30 mL
Milk	1 1/2 cups	375 mL
Grated smoked Gouda cheese	1 cup	250 mL
Onion powder	3/4 tsp.	4 mL
Pepper	1/4 tsp.	1 mL
Thinly sliced unpeeled baking potato	4 cups	1 L
Grated Parmesan cheese	1/2 cup	125 mL

BEFORE: *1 serving:*
456 Calories; **34 g Total Fat** *(21 g Sat);*
781 mg Sodium

AFTER: *1 serving:*
199 Calories; **6 g Total Fat** *(0 g Mono, 0 g Poly, 3.5 g Sat);*
21 mg Cholesterol;
27 g Carbohydrate;
2 g Fibre; 9 g Protein;
330 mg Sodium

Whisk broth and flour in large saucepan until smooth. Whisk in milk. Cook on medium, stirring occasionally, until boiling and slightly thickened.

Add next 3 ingredients. Remove from heat. Stir until Gouda cheese is melted.

Add potato. Stir to coat. Spoon into greased 2 quart (2 L) casserole.

Sprinkle with Parmesan cheese. Bake, covered, in 350°F (175°C) oven for about 1 hour until potato is tender. Remove cover. Bake for about 20 minutes until golden. Serves 6.

Pictured on page 125.

Paré Pointer

A nail and a boxer are very different. A nail gets knocked in.
A boxer gets knocked out.

Lemon Basil Vinaigrette

Traditional vinaigrettes use a 3:1 ratio of oil to acid. This makeover reduces the oil and fat but still delivers plenty of punchy flavour with aromatic ingredients such as lemon and basil.

Olive oil	1/4 cup	60 mL
Water	1/4 cup	60 mL
Lemon juice	3 tbsp.	50 mL
Finely shredded basil	1 tbsp.	15 mL
Liquid honey	1 tbsp.	15 mL
Dijon mustard	2 tsp.	10 mL
Grated lemon zest (see Tip, page 151)	1 tsp.	5 mL
Salt	1/8 tsp.	0.5 mL
Pepper	1/4 tsp.	1 mL

Whisk all 9 ingredients in small bowl. Makes about 3/4 cup (175 mL).

BEFORE: *2 tbsp. (30 mL): 180 Calories;* **19.7 g Total Fat** *(2.7 g Sat); 74 mg Sodium*

AFTER: *2 tbsp. (30 mL): 97 Calories;* **9 g Total Fat** *(7 g Mono, 1 g Poly, 1.5 g Sat); 0 mg Cholesterol; 4 g Carbohydrate; 0 g Fibre; 0 g Protein; 73 mg Sodium*

Simply Fresh Salsa

Simply good for you! Serve with tortilla chips, or use as a low-calorie condiment on burgers, tacos or grilled fish.

Diced seeded Roma (plum) tomato	2 cups	500 mL
Finely chopped yellow pepper	1/2 cup	125 mL
Finely chopped red onion	1/4 cup	60 mL
Chopped fresh cilantro (or parsley)	2 tbsp.	30 mL
Lime juice	1 tbsp.	15 mL
Finely chopped fresh jalapeño pepper (see Tip, page 13)	2 tsp.	10 mL
Garlic clove, minced (or 1/4 tsp., 1 mL, powder)	1	1
Grated lime zest (see Tip, page 151)	1 tsp.	5 mL
Ground cumin	1/2 tsp.	2 mL
Salt	1/4 tsp.	1 mL
Pepper	1/8 tsp.	0.5 mL

(continued on next page)

Combine all 11 ingredients in medium bowl. Let stand at room temperature for 1 hour to blend flavours. Makes about 2 cups (500 mL).

Pictured on page 72 and on back cover.

BEFORE: *1/4 cup (60 mL): 25 Calories; 0 g Total Fat (0 g Sat);* **440 mg Sodium**

AFTER: *1/4 cup (60 mL): 14 Calories; 0 g Total Fat (0 g Mono, 0 g Poly, 0 g Sat); 0 mg Cholesterol; 3 g Carbohydrate; 1 g Fibre; 1 g Protein;* **76 mg Sodium**

Citrus Sesame Dressing

This amber dressing features flavourful notes of lemon, lime and orange. Very good with fresh celery, carrot and broccoli. Could also be drizzled over shrimp or salmon.

Orange juice	1 cup	250 mL
Lemon juice	2 tbsp.	30 mL
Lime juice	2 tbsp.	30 mL
Maple syrup	1 tbsp.	15 mL
Sesame oil (for flavour)	1 tbsp.	15 mL
Soy sauce	1 tbsp.	15 mL
Finely grated ginger root (or 1/2 tsp., 2 mL, ground ginger)	2 tsp.	10 mL
Grated lemon zest (see Tip, page 151)	1/4 tsp.	1 mL
Grated lime zest (see Tip, page 151)	1/4 tsp.	1 mL
Pepper	1/4 tsp.	1 mL

Bring orange juice to a boil in small saucepan. Reduce heat to medium. Boil gently, uncovered, for about 20 minutes, stirring occasionally, until reduced to 1/4 cup (60 mL). Transfer to small bowl. Cool. Transfer to blender.

Add remaining 9 ingredients. Process until smooth. Makes about 3/4 cup (175 mL).

BEFORE: *2 tbsp. (30 mL): 90 Calories;* **8.6 g Total Fat** *(1 g Sat); 250 mg Sodium*

AFTER: *2 tbsp. (30 mL): 53 Calories;* **2 g Total Fat** *(1 g Mono, 1 g Poly, 0 g Sat); 0 mg Cholesterol; 7 g Carbohydrate; 0 g Fibre; 0 g Protein; 160 mg Sodium*

Spicy Peanut Sauce

A versatile sauce that can be used in stir-fries, on pasta, or as a barbecue sauce or dipping sauce. Kidney beans add fibre and protein, and fresh peanuts add less sugar and sodium than peanut butter.

Canned white kidney beans, rinsed and drained	1 cup	250 mL
Unsalted peanuts	1 cup	250 mL
Brown sugar, packed	1/2 cup	125 mL
Water	1/4 cup	60 mL
Low-sodium soy sauce	3 tbsp.	50 mL
Rice vinegar	3 tbsp.	50 mL
Finely grated ginger root (or 1 1/2 tsp., 7 mL, ground ginger)	2 tbsp.	30 mL
Roasted sesame seeds	2 tbsp.	30 mL
Chili paste (sambal oelek)	2 tsp.	10 mL
Garlic powder	1 tsp.	5 mL

Process all 10 ingredients in food processor until smooth. Makes about 2 1/4 cups (550 mL).

BEFORE: *2 tbsp. (30 mL): 120 Calories; 9 g Total Fat (3 g Sat);* ***339 mg Sodium***

AFTER: *2 tbsp. (30 mL): 86 Calories; 4 g Total Fat (2 g Mono, 1.5 g Poly, 0.5 g Sat); 0 mg Cholesterol; 10 g Carbohydrate; 1 g Fibre; 3 g Protein;* ***127 mg Sodium***

Creamy Herb Dressing

This refreshing dressing announces that summer has arrived! Goes particularly well with leafy greens, or try it on your next potato salad.

1% buttermilk	1/2 cup	125 mL
Finely chopped green onion (white part only)	1 tbsp.	15 mL
Mayonnaise	1 tbsp.	15 mL
White wine vinegar	1 tbsp.	15 mL
Chopped fresh dill (or 1/2 tsp., 2 mL, dried)	2 tsp.	10 mL
Chopped fresh parsley (or 1/2 tsp., 2 mL, flakes)	2 tsp.	10 mL
Granulated sugar	1/2 tsp.	2 mL

(continued on next page)

Whisk all 7 ingredients in small bowl. Makes about 3/4 cup (175 mL).

BEFORE: *2 tbsp. (30 mL):* **100 Calories**; *10 g Total Fat (2 g Sat); 270 mg Sodium*

AFTER: *2 tbsp. (30 mL):* **28 Calories**; *2 g Total Fat (0 g Mono, 0 g Poly, 0 g Sat); 3 mg Cholesterol; 1 g Carbohydrate; 0 g Fibre; 0 g Protein; 32 mg Sodium*

Roasted Vegetable Sauce

Satisfy your sweet tooth with a helping of naturally sweet roasted vegetables. This versatile sauce goes great with pasta, chicken or seafood. Store in an airtight container in the refrigerator for up to five days or in the freezer for up to six months.

Olive oil	1 tbsp.	15 mL
Small onions, chopped	2	2
Garlic cloves, peeled	4	4
Roma (plum) tomatoes, halved lengthwise	2 1/2 lbs.	1.1 kg
Medium red peppers, halved	2	2
Balsamic vinegar	2 tbsp.	30 mL
Tomato paste (see Tip, page 32)	2 tbsp.	30 mL
Granulated sugar	2 tsp.	10 mL
Dried oregano	1 tsp.	5 mL
Salt	1/2 tsp.	2 mL
Pepper	1/2 tsp.	2 mL

Toss first 4 ingredients in large bowl until coated. Spread on greased large baking sheet with sides. Place red pepper on same baking sheet. Bake in 450°F (230°C) oven for about 45 minutes, stirring once at halftime, until vegetables are tender. Let stand for 10 minutes. Transfer vegetables and any liquid to food processor. Carefully process until smooth (see Safety Tip). Transfer to large saucepan.

Add remaining 6 ingredients. Stir. Bring to a boil. Reduce heat to medium-low. Simmer, partially covered, for 10 minutes to blend flavours. Makes about 5 cups (1.25 L).

Safety Tip: Follow manufacturer's instructions for processing hot liquids.

BEFORE: *1/2 cup (125 mL): 80 Calories; 2 g Total Fat (0 g Sat);* **540 mg Sodium**

AFTER: *1/2 cup (125 mL): 68 Calories; 2 g Total Fat (1 g Mono, 0 g Poly, 0 g Sat); 0 mg Cholesterol; 13 g Carbohydrate; 3 g Fibre; 2 g Protein;* **134 mg Sodium**

Roasted Garlic Cheese Sauce

Roasted garlic adds plenty of flavour to this smooth, creamy cheese sauce.
Goes perfectly with broccoli, asparagus or pasta.

Small garlic bulb	1	1
Olive oil	1 tsp.	5 mL
All-purpose flour	2 tbsp.	30 mL
Prepared vegetable broth	1/2 cup	125 mL
Skim milk	1 1/2 cups	375 mL
Soft goat (chèvre) cheese, cut up	4 oz.	113 g
Crumbled light feta cheese	1/3 cup	75 mL

Trim 1/4 inch (6 mm) from garlic bulb to expose tops of cloves, leaving bulb intact. Drizzle cut end with olive oil. Wrap loosely in greased foil. Bake in 375°F (190°C) oven for about 45 minutes until tender. Let stand until cool enough to handle. Squeeze garlic bulb to remove cloves from skin. Mash. Discard skin. Transfer mashed garlic to medium saucepan.

Add flour and broth. Whisk until smooth. Whisk in milk. Cook on medium, stirring occasionally, until boiling and slightly thickened. Remove from heat.

Whisk in goat and feta cheese until melted. Carefully process with hand blender or in blender until smooth (see Safety Tip). Makes about 2 1/2 cups (625 mL).

Safety Tip: Follow manufacturer's instructions for processing hot liquids.

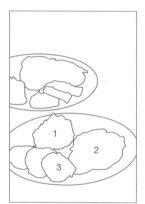

1. Broccoflower Bake, page 118
2. Smoky Cheese Potato Scallop, page 119
3. Whiskey Glazed Tenderloin, page 88

BEFORE: *2 tbsp. (30 mL):* **66 Calories**; *5 g Total Fat (3 g Sat); 106 mg Sodium*

AFTER: *2 tbsp. (30 mL):* **35 Calories**; *2 g Total Fat (0 g Mono, 0 g Poly, 1 g Sat); 4 mg Cholesterol; 3 g Carbohydrate; 0 g Fibre; 2 g Protein; 74 mg Sodium*

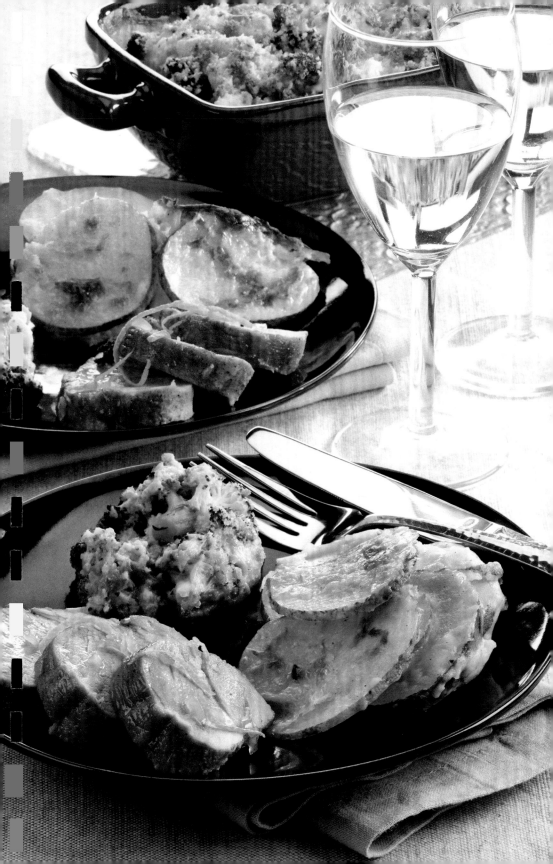

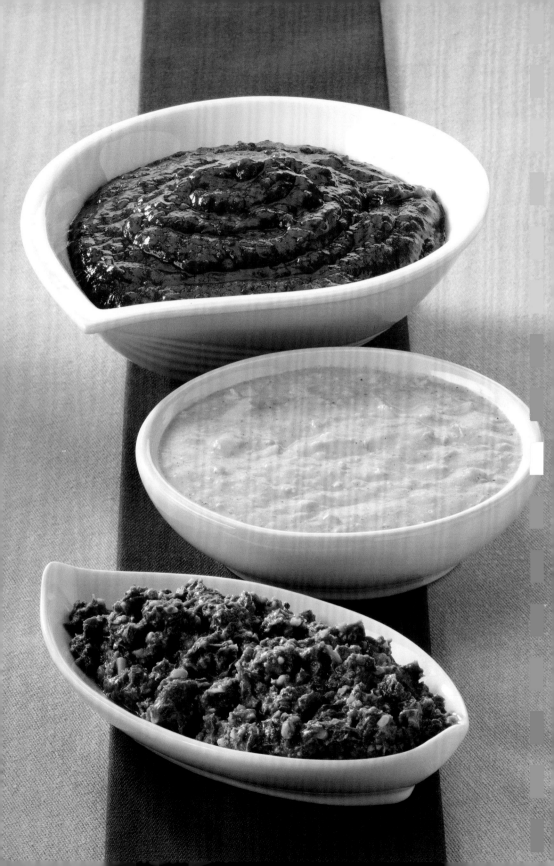

Coconut Curry Sauce

Enjoy the sweetness of coconut and the heat of curry in this sauce that's perfect for serving with grilled chicken, seafood or pork.

Canola oil	1/2 tsp.	2 mL
Finely chopped onion	1/2 cup	125 mL
Medium sweetened coconut	1/4 cup	60 mL
Garlic cloves, minced (or 1/2 tsp., 2 mL, powder)	2	2
Hot curry powder	1 tbsp.	15 mL
All-purpose flour	2 tbsp.	30 mL
Can of light coconut milk	14 oz.	398 mL
Apple juice	1/4 cup	60 mL
Brown sugar, packed	1 tbsp.	15 mL
Finely grated ginger root (or 3/4 tsp., 4 mL, ground ginger)	1 tbsp.	15 mL
Lime juice	1 tbsp.	15 mL
Salt	1/2 tsp.	2 mL
Pepper	1/4 tsp.	1 mL

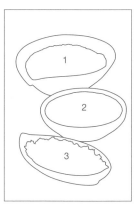

1. Cranberry Chipotle BBQ Sauce, page 128
2. Coconut Curry Sauce, above
3. Basil Spinach Pesto, page 129

Props: Moderno

Heat canola oil in small saucepan on medium. Add next 4 ingredients. Cook for about 5 minutes, stirring often, until onion is softened. Sprinkle with flour. Heat and stir for 1 minute.

Slowly add coconut milk, stirring constantly until smooth. Add remaining 6 ingredients. Heat and stir until boiling and thickened. Makes about 2 cups (500 mL).

Pictured at left.

BEFORE: *2 tbsp (30 mL):* **110 Calories**; *8 g Total Fat (6 g Sat); 190 mg Sodium*

AFTER: *2 tbsp (30 mL):* **43 Calories**; *2.5 g Total Fat (0 g Mono, 0 g Poly, 2 g Sat); 0 mg Cholesterol; 4 g Carbohydrate; 0 g Fibre; 0 g Protein; 84 mg Sodium*

Cranberry Chipotle BBQ Sauce

Homemade barbecue sauce that is lower in sodium and doubles as a dipping sauce. Mildly sweet with some tangy notes, followed by some smoky chili heat. Cranberries are high in antioxidants.

Fresh (or frozen, thawed) cranberries	2 cups	500 mL
Chopped onion	1 cup	250 mL
Tomato sauce	1 cup	250 mL
Brown sugar, packed	1/2 cup	125 mL
Orange juice	1/2 cup	125 mL
Soy sauce	3 tbsp.	50 mL
Finely chopped chipotle peppers in adobo sauce (see Tip, below)	2 tbsp.	30 mL
Dry mustard	1 tbsp.	15 mL
Garlic cloves, chopped (or 3/4 tsp., 4 mL, powder)	3	3
Pepper	1/2 tsp.	2 mL

BEFORE: *2 tbsp. (30 mL):*
50 Calories; 0.5 g Total Fat
(0 g Sat); ***520 mg Sodium***

AFTER: *2 tbsp. (30 mL):*
40 Calories; 1 g Total Fat
(0 g Mono, 0 g Poly,
0 g Sat); 0 mg Cholesterol;
9 g Carbohydrate;
1 g Fibre; 1 g Protein;
230 mg Sodium

Combine all 10 ingredients in large saucepan. Bring to a boil. Reduce heat to medium-low. Boil gently, uncovered, for about 15 minutes, stirring occasionally, until cranberries are softened. Carefully process with hand blender or in blender until smooth (see Safety Tip). Bring to a boil. Boil gently, uncovered, for about 10 minutes, stirring often, until thickened. Makes about 2 1/3 cups (575 mL).

Pictured on page 126.

Safety Tip: Follow manufacturer's instructions for processing hot liquids.

 tip Chipotle chili peppers are smoked jalapeño peppers. Be sure to wash your hands after handling. To store any leftover chipotle chili peppers, divide into recipe-friendly portions and freeze, with sauce, in airtight containers for up to one year.

Basil Spinach Pesto

Try this delicious, low-fat pesto tossed with pasta, sautéed shrimp or tomato salad, or sprinkled over chicken or tomato soup. Store pesto in the refrigerator for up to five days or in the freezer for up to three months.

Fresh basil leaves, lightly packed	2 cups	500 mL
Fresh spinach leaves, lightly packed	2 cups	500 mL
Fresh parsley leaves, lightly packed	1 cup	250 mL
Olive (or canola) oil	1/4 cup	60 mL
Walnuts, toasted (see Tip, page 110)	1/4 cup	60 mL
Grated Parmesan cheese	3 tbsp.	50 mL
White wine vinegar	2 tbsp.	30 mL
Garlic cloves, minced	2	2
Salt	1/4 tsp.	1 mL
Pepper	1/4 tsp.	1 mL

BEFORE: *1 tbsp. (15 mL):*
62 Calories; **6.5 g Total Fat** *(1.1 g Sat);*
49 mg Sodium

AFTER: *1 tbsp. (15 mL):*
35 Calories; **3.5 g Total Fat** *(2 g Mono, 1 g Poly, 0.5 g Sat); 1 mg Cholesterol; 1 g Carbohydrate; 0 g Fibre; 1 g Protein; 44 mg Sodium*

Process all 10 ingredients in food processor, scraping down sides if necessary, until smooth. Fill small clean plastic containers to within 1/2 inch (12 mm) of top (see Tip, below). Wipe rims. Cover with tight-fitting lids. Makes about 1 1/3 cups (325 mL).

Pictured on page 126.

 When using plastic containers for freezing preserves, select containers without any cracks or leaks. Plastic freezer jars designed to store preserves in the freezer are also available at many grocery stores.

Strawberry Rhubarb Turnovers

Delicious strawberry-rhubarb filling hides inside these crispy cinnamon-sugar turnovers. Flour tortillas make a much lower-fat alternative to pastry.

Chopped fresh (or frozen, thawed) rhubarb	1 1/2 cups	375 mL
Granulated sugar	2/3 cup	150 mL
All-purpose flour	3 tbsp.	50 mL
Chopped fresh strawberries	1 cup	250 mL
Lemon juice	2 tsp.	10 mL
Flour tortillas (7 1/2 inch, 19 cm, diameter)	6	6
Cooking spray		
Granulated sugar	1/4 cup	60 mL
Ground cinnamon	1 1/2 tsp.	7 mL

BEFORE: *1 turnover:*
461 Calories; **26 g Total Fat** *(7 g Sat);*
206 mg Sodium

AFTER: *1 turnover:*
287 Calories; **3 g Total Fat** *(1.5 g Mono, 0.5 g Poly, 1 g Sat); 0 mg Cholesterol; 61 g Carbohydrate; 3 g Fibre; 5 g Protein; 215 mg Sodium*

Combine rhubarb and first amount of sugar in 2 quart (2 L) casserole. Microwave, covered, on high (100%) for about 5 minutes, stirring at halftime, until rhubarb is softened (see Tip, below). Whisk in flour. Microwave, covered, on high (100%) for about 3 minutes until mixture is thickened.

Add strawberries and lemon juice. Stir.

Spoon about 1/4 cup (60 mL) rhubarb mixture along centre of tortilla. Fold sides over filling. Roll up tightly from bottom to enclose. Secure with wooden pick. Spray with cooking spray.

Combine second amount of sugar and cinnamon in shallow bowl. Roll filled tortilla in sugar mixture. Place, seam-side down, on greased baking sheet with sides. Repeat with remaining rhubarb mixture, tortillas, cooking spray and sugar mixture. Spray rolls with cooking spray. Cut several small vents in top of rolls to allow steam to escape. Bake in 450°F (230°C) oven for about 10 minutes until golden and crisp. Makes 6 turnovers.

tip The microwaves used in our test kitchen are 900 watts—but microwaves are sold in many different powers. You should be able to find the wattage of yours by opening the door and looking for the mandatory label. If your microwave is more than 900 watts, you may need to reduce the cooking time. If it's less than 900 watts, you'll probably need to increase the cooking time.

Apricot Brownie Bites

Chocolate seems to make any day better! These low-fat brownies boast lots of rich chocolate flavour.

Granulated sugar	3/4 cup	175 mL
All-purpose flour	2/3 cup	150 mL
Cocoa, sifted if lumpy	1/2 cup	125 mL
Baking powder	1 tsp.	5 mL
Salt	1/4 tsp.	1 mL
Chopped dried apricot	2/3 cup	150 mL
Water	1/3 cup	75 mL
Semi-sweet chocolate baking squares (1 oz., 28 g, each), chopped	2	2
Butter	3 tbsp.	50 mL
Water	1/4 cup	60 mL
Egg whites (large)	2	2
Large egg, fork-beaten	1	1

BEFORE: *1 brownie:*
154 Calories; *7.4 g Total Fat (3.1 g Sat); 76 mg Sodium*

AFTER: *1 brownie:*
80 Calories; *2.5 g Total Fat (0.5 g Mono, 0 g Poly, 1.5 g Sat);*
10 mg Cholesterol;
14 g Carbohydrate;
1 g Fibre; 2 g Protein;
54 mg Sodium

Combine first 5 ingredients in large bowl. Make a well in centre.

Bring apricot and first amount of water to a boil in small saucepan. Reduce heat to medium-low. Cook, covered, for about 10 minutes until apricot is softened. Transfer to food processor. Carefully process until smooth (see Safety Tip).

Put chocolate and butter into microwave-safe small bowl. Microwave on medium (50%) for about 90 seconds, stirring every 20 seconds, until almost melted (see Tip, page 130). Stir until smooth. Add to apricot.

Add remaining 3 ingredients. Carefully process until smooth. Add to flour mixture. Stir until just moistened. Fill 24 greased mini muffin cups 3/4 full. Bake in 350°F (175°C) oven for about 14 minutes until wooden pick inserted in centre of brownie comes out moist but not wet with batter. Do not overbake. Let stand in pan for 5 minutes before removing to wire rack to cool. Makes 24 brownies.

Safety Tip: Follow manufacturer's instructions for processing hot liquids.

Plus Minus Carrot Cake

A traditional carrot cake—plus a healthy dose of banana and zucchini, and minus much of the oil used in most carrot cake recipes.

All-purpose flour	1 1/2 cups	375 mL
Whole-wheat flour	1 cup	250 mL
Baking powder	1 1/2 tsp.	7 mL
Baking soda	1 tsp.	5 mL
Ground cinnamon	1 tsp.	5 mL
Ground cardamom	1/2 tsp.	2 mL
Ground cloves	1/8 tsp.	0.5 mL
Salt	1/4 tsp.	1 mL
Egg whites (large)	2	2
Large eggs	2	2
Granulated sugar	1 cup	250 mL
Brown sugar, packed	3/4 cup	175 mL
Canola oil	2/3 cup	150 mL
Mashed ripe banana	2/3 cup	150 mL
Grated carrot	2 cups	500 mL
Grated zucchini (with peel), squeezed dry	1 cup	250 mL
Icing (confectioner's) sugar	1/2 cup	125 mL
95% fat-free spreadable cream cheese	3 tbsp.	50 mL
Lemon juice	1 tsp.	5 mL

BEFORE: *1 slice:*
425 Calories; **23 g Total Fat** *(4 g Sat); 260 mg Sodium*

AFTER: *1 slice:*
279 Calories; **10 g Total Fat** *(6 g Mono, 2.5 g Poly, 1 g Sat); 18 mg Cholesterol; 45 g Carbohydrate; 2 g Fibre; 4 g Protein; 189 mg Sodium*

Combine first 8 ingredients in medium bowl.

Beat next 6 ingredients in large bowl until smooth. Add flour mixture in 2 additions, stirring after each addition until no dry flour remains.

Add carrot and zucchini. Stir until just combined. Pour into greased 10 cup (2.5 L) bundt pan. Bake in 350°F (175°C) oven for about 55 minutes until wooden pick inserted in centre of cake comes out clean. Let stand in pan on wire rack for 10 minutes. Invert onto wire rack to cool completely.

Beat remaining 3 ingredients in small bowl until mixture is smooth and barely pourable. Spread over cake. Let stand for 10 minutes. Cuts into 16 slices.

Mango Nut Upside-Down Cake

When you flip the cake over, you discover a pleasantly sweet mango and macadamia topping.

Brown sugar, packed	1/4 cup	60 mL
Butter, softened	1 tbsp.	15 mL
Diced fresh (or frozen, thawed) mango	1 1/2 cups	375 mL
Macadamia nuts, toasted (see Tip, page 110) and chopped	1/4 cup	60 mL
Egg whites (large)	3	3
Cream of tartar	1/2 tsp.	2 mL
Brown sugar, packed	1/2 cup	125 mL
1% buttermilk (or soured milk, see Tip, page 136)	1/2 cup	125 mL
Unsweetened applesauce	1/2 cup	125 mL
Butter, softened	2 tbsp.	30 mL
Canola oil	2 tbsp.	30 mL
All-purpose flour	1 1/2 cups	375 mL
Baking powder	1 tsp.	5 mL
Baking soda	1/4 tsp.	1 mL
Salt	1/2 tsp.	2 mL

BEFORE: *1 piece:*
391 Calories; **22.2 g Total** *Fat (7.9 g Sat); 482 mg Sodium*

AFTER: *1 piece:*
267 Calories; **10 g Total Fat** *(5 g Mono, 1 g Poly, 3 g Sat); 12 mg Cholesterol; 41 g Carbohydrate; 1 g Fibre; 4 g Protein; 217 mg Sodium*

Combine first amounts of brown sugar and butter in 9 x 9 inch (23 x 23 cm) pan. Bake in 350°F (175°C) oven for about 5 minutes, stirring at halftime, until sugar is melted and starts to bubble.

Scatter mango and nuts over top. Set aside.

Beat egg whites and cream of tartar in medium bowl until stiff peaks form.

Beat next 5 ingredients in large bowl until smooth.

Combine remaining 4 ingredients in small bowl. Add to buttermilk mixture. Beat on low until just combined. Fold in egg white mixture until no white streaks remain. Spread over mango mixture. Bake in 350°F (175°C) oven for about 40 minutes until wooden pick inserted in centre of cake comes out clean. Let stand on wire rack for 5 minutes. Invert onto serving plate. Cuts into 9 pieces.

Spiced Vanilla Pound Cake

A very moist cake with a comforting old-fashioned feel—and it's low in fat, too.
Dust with icing sugar if desired.

All-purpose flour	3 cups	750 mL
Baking powder	2 tsp.	10 mL
Baking soda	3/4 tsp.	4 mL
Ground cinnamon	1 tsp.	5 mL
Ground ginger	1 tsp.	5 mL
Salt	1/2 tsp.	2 mL
Ground cloves	1/8 tsp.	0.5 mL
Egg whites (large)	3	3
Low-fat vanilla yogurt	2 cups	500 mL
Brown sugar, packed	1 cup	250 mL
Granulated sugar	1/2 cup	125 mL
Butter, melted	1/4 cup	60 mL
Canola oil	1/4 cup	60 mL
Egg yolks (large)	3	3
Apple cider vinegar	1 tbsp.	15 mL
Vanilla extract	1 tbsp.	15 mL

BEFORE: *1 slice:*
554 Calories; *25.6 g Total Fat (12 g Sat); 346 mg Sodium*

AFTER: *1 slice:*
258 Calories; *8 g Total Fat (3 g Mono, 1 g Poly, 2.5 g Sat); 49 mg Cholesterol; 42 g Carbohydrate; 1 g Fibre; 5 g Protein; 225 mg Sodium*

Combine first 7 ingredients in medium bowl.

Beat egg whites in small bowl until stiff peaks form.

Beat remaining 8 ingredients in large bowl until smooth. Add flour mixture. Stir until just combined. Fold in egg whites. Spread in greased 10 cup (2.5 L) bundt pan. Bake in 350°F (175°C) oven for about 45 minutes until wooden pick inserted in centre of cake comes out clean. Let stand in pan for 10 minutes. Invert onto wire rack to cool. Cuts into 16 slices.

Peanut Butter Oatmeal Cookies

Pass the cold milk, please! A snack-time favourite updated with less fat. If you already have smooth peanut butter in the pantry, just add a tablespoon or two of chopped unsalted peanuts.

All-purpose flour	1 1/2 cups	375 mL
Quick-cooking rolled oats	1 1/3 cups	325 mL
Wheat germ, toasted (see Tip, page 105)	1/3 cup	75 mL
Baking soda	1/2 tsp.	2 mL
Salt	1/2 tsp.	2 mL
Brown sugar, packed	1 1/4 cups	300 mL
Butter, melted	1/2 cup	125 mL
Crunchy peanut butter	1/2 cup	125 mL
Large eggs	2	2
Vanilla extract	1 tsp.	5 mL

BEFORE: *2 cookies:*
***376 Calories**; 22 g Total Fat (8 g Sat); 240 mg Sodium*

AFTER: *2 cookies:*
***200 Calories**; 10 g Total Fat (2 g Mono, 0 g Poly, 4 g Sat); 28 mg Cholesterol; 28 g Carbohydrate; 2 g Fibre; 4 g Protein; 160 mg Sodium*

Combine first 5 ingredients in medium bowl.

Beat remaining 5 ingredients in large bowl until smooth. Add flour mixture. Mix until no dry flour remains. Roll into balls, using about 1 tbsp. (15 mL) for each. Arrange balls, about 2 1/2 inches (6.4 cm) apart, on greased cookie sheets. Flatten slightly with fork. Bake in 350°F (175°C) oven for about 10 minutes until golden. Let stand on cookie sheets for 5 minutes before removing to wire racks to cool. Makes about 38 cookies.

Fruitfull Bran Muffins

Everyone knows that bran muffins are supposed to be good for you, but often they're surprisingly high in fat and sugar. This low-fat update adds sweet bites of cranberries and apricots and a nice crunch from pumpkin seeds and flaxseed.

1% buttermilk (or soured milk, see Tip, below)	1 cup	250 mL
Natural wheat bran	1 cup	250 mL
Large egg	1	1
Brown sugar, packed	1/2 cup	125 mL
Canola oil	1/4 cup	60 mL
Fancy (mild) molasses	1/4 cup	60 mL
Whole-wheat flour	1 1/4 cups	300 mL
Flaxseed	2 tbsp.	30 mL
Baking powder	1 1/2 tsp.	7 mL
Baking soda	1/2 tsp.	2 mL
Salt	1/2 tsp.	2 mL
Dried cranberries, chopped	1/3 cup	75 mL
Finely chopped dried apricot	1/3 cup	75 mL
Raw pumpkin seeds, toasted (see Tip, page 110) and chopped	1/3 cup	75 mL

BEFORE: *1 muffin:*
293 Calories; *12 g Total Fat (6 g Sat); 253 mg Sodium*

AFTER: *1 muffin:*
196 Calories; *6 g Total Fat (3 g Mono, 1.5 g Poly, 0.5 g Sat); 14 mg Cholesterol; 33 g Carbohydrate; 4 g Fibre; 4 g Protein; 221 mg Sodium*

Stir buttermilk into bran in large bowl. Let stand for 10 minutes.

Add next 4 ingredients. Beat well.

Combine next 5 ingredients in small bowl. Add to bran mixture.

Add remaining 3 ingredients. Stir until just moistened. Fill 12 greased muffin cups 3/4 full. Bake in 375°F (190°C) oven for about 20 minutes until wooden pick inserted in centre of muffin comes out clean. Let stand in pan for 5 minutes before removing to wire rack to cool. Makes 12 muffins.

 tip

To make soured milk, measure 1 tbsp. (15 mL) white vinegar or lemon juice into a 1 cup (250 mL) liquid measure. Add enough milk to make 1 cup (250 mL). Stir. Let stand for 1 minute.

Blueberry Oatmeal Muffins

Instead of giving in to that fatty blueberry muffin at the bakery, make your own and add some healthier ingredients. This remake is boosted with fibre-rich oats, low-fat yogurt and applesauce.

Large flake rolled oats	1 cup	250 mL
Low-fat vanilla yogurt	1 cup	250 mL
Grated lemon zest (see Tip, page 151)	2 tsp.	10 mL
Large eggs	2	2
Unsweetened applesauce	1/2 cup	125 mL
Canola oil	3 tbsp.	50 mL
Lemon juice	1 tbsp.	15 mL
All-purpose flour	1 1/2 cups	375 mL
Brown sugar, packed	2/3 cup	150 mL
Baking powder	2 tsp.	10 mL
Ground cinnamon	1 tsp.	5 mL
Baking soda	1/2 tsp.	2 mL
Salt	1/2 tsp.	2 mL
Fresh (or frozen) blueberries	1 1/2 cups	375 mL

BEFORE: *1 muffin:*
308 Calories; 13 g Total Fat
*(**8 g Sat**); 274 mg Sodium*

AFTER: *1 muffin:*
205 Calories; 5 g Total Fat
(2.5 g Mono, 1.5 g Poly,
***0.5 g Sat**);*
25 mg Cholesterol;
36 g Carbohydrate;
2 g Fibre; 4 g Protein;
220 mg Sodium

Combine first 3 ingredients in medium bowl. Let stand for 10 minutes.

Add next 4 ingredients. Mix well.

Combine next 6 ingredients in large bowl. Make a well in centre.

Add blueberries and rolled oat mixture. Stir until just moistened. Fill 12 greased muffin cups 3/4 full. Bake in 375°F (190°C) oven for about 22 minutes until wooden pick inserted in centre of muffin comes out clean. Let stand in pan for 5 minutes before removing to wire rack to cool. Makes 12 muffins.

Paré Pointer

A dressmaker cuts dresses and a nurse dresses cuts.

Mango Peach Pie

A very pretty pie with a ginger-accented fruit filling. The crust uses canola oil,
which helps to drastically reduce the amount of saturated fat.

WHOLE-WHEAT PASTRY

Whole-wheat flour	2 1/2 cups	625 mL
Granulated sugar	1 tbsp.	15 mL
Salt	1/8 tsp.	0.5 mL
Cold butter, cut up	1/3 cup	75 mL
Canola oil	1/3 cup	75 mL
Ice water	1/3 cup	75 mL

MANGO PEACH FILLING

Cans of sliced peaches in juice (14 oz., 398 mL, each), drained	2	2
Frozen mango pieces, thawed and drained	3 cups	750 mL
Brown sugar, packed	1/3 cup	75 mL
Ginger marmalade	1/3 cup	75 mL
Minute tapioca	2 tbsp.	30 mL
Large egg, fork-beaten	1	1

BEFORE: *1 wedge:*
610 Calories; 35 g Total Fat
*(**15 g Sat**); 3 g Fibre;*
356 mg Sodium

AFTER: *1 wedge:*
446 Calories; 18 g Total
Fat (8 g Mono, 3 g Poly,
***6 g Sat**);*
27 mg Cholesterol;
69 g Carbohydrate;
6 g Fibre; 6 g Protein;
119 mg Sodium

Whole-Wheat Pastry: Combine first 3 ingredients in large bowl. Cut in butter until mixture resembles coarse crumbs. Add canola oil. Toss with fork to combine.

Slowly add water, stirring with fork until mixture starts to come together. Do not overmix. Turn out pastry onto work surface. Shape into slightly flattened disc. Wrap with plastic wrap. Chill for 30 minutes. Divide pastry into 2 portions, making 1 portion slightly larger than the other. Roll out larger portion on lightly floured surface to about 1/8 inch (3 mm) thickness. Line 9 inch (23 cm) pie plate.

Mango Peach Filling: Combine first 5 ingredients in medium bowl. Fill pie shell. Roll remaining pastry on lightly floured surface to about 1/8 inch (3 mm) thickness.

(continued on next page)

Brush edge of bottom pie shell with egg. Cover with remaining pastry. Trim and crimp decorative edge to seal. Brush with remaining egg. Cut several small vents in top of pastry to allow steam to escape. Bake on bottom rack in 425°F (220°C) oven for 15 minutes. Reduce heat to 375°F (190°C). Bake for about 40 minutes until pastry is golden. Cuts into 8 wedges.

Pictured on page 143.

Chocolate Chip Cookies

Whole-wheat flour and canola oil add healthier elements to the ever-popular chocolate chip cookie. Another trick? Use mini chocolate chips—they distribute nicely through the cookies, so you can use less and still get lots of chocolate taste!

All-purpose flour	1 1/4 cups	300 mL
Whole-wheat flour	1 cup	250 mL
Baking soda	1/2 tsp.	2 mL
Salt	1/4 tsp.	1 mL
Large eggs	2	2
Brown sugar, packed	1 1/4 cups	300 mL
Butter, melted	1/4 cup	60 mL
Canola oil	3 tbsp.	50 mL
Vanilla extract	1 tsp.	5 mL
Mini semi-sweet chocolate chips	1 1/2 cups	375 mL

BEFORE: *2 cookies:*
306 Calories; **17 g Total Fat** *(8 g Sat);*
196 mg Sodium

AFTER: *2 cookies:*
210 Calories; **9 g Total Fat** *(2 g Mono, 0.5 g Poly, 4 g Sat); 21 mg Cholesterol; 30 g Carbohydrate; 1 g Fibre; 3 g Protein; 92 mg Sodium*

Combine first 4 ingredients in small bowl.

Beat next 5 ingredients in large bowl until smooth. Add flour mixture. Mix until no dry flour remains.

Add chocolate chips. Mix well. Drop, using about 1 tbsp. (15 mL) for each cookie, about 2 inches (5 cm) apart onto greased cookie sheets. Flatten slightly with fork. Bake in 350°F (175°C) oven for about 10 minutes until golden. Let stand on cookie sheets for 5 minutes before removing to wire racks to cool. Makes about 46 cookies.

Pictured on page 143.

Double Chocolate Cupcakes

These lower-fat cupcakes are sure to be a hit at your next picnic or party!
The chocolate cream cheese icing has just the right dose of sweetness.

1% buttermilk (or soured milk, see Tip, page 136)	1 cup	250 mL
Canola oil	6 tbsp.	100 mL
Egg whites (large)	2	2
Large egg	1	1
Vanilla extract	1 tsp.	5 mL
All-purpose flour	1 1/2 cups	375 mL
Granulated sugar	1 cup	250 mL
Cocoa, sifted if lumpy	1/2 cup	125 mL
Baking powder	1 1/2 tsp.	7 mL
Baking soda	1/2 tsp.	2 mL
Salt	1/4 tsp.	1 mL
95% fat-free spreadable cream cheese	1/2 cup	125 mL
Butter, softened	2 tbsp.	30 mL
Icing (confectioner's) sugar	2 cups	500 mL
Cocoa, sifted if lumpy	1/3 cup	75 mL

BEFORE: *1 cupcake:*
362 Calories; 18 g Total Fat
*(**11 g Sat**); 307 mg Sodium*

AFTER: *1 cupcake:*
308 Calories; 11 g Total Fat
(5 g Mono, 2 g Poly,
***2.5 g Sat**);*
22 mg Cholesterol;
50 g Carbohydrate;
2 g Fibre; 5 g Protein;
250 mg Sodium

Beat first 5 ingredients in large bowl until smooth.

Combine next 6 ingredients in medium bowl. Add to buttermilk mixture. Beat until just combined. Fill 12 paper-lined muffin cups 3/4 full. Bake in 350°F (175°C) oven for about 18 minutes until wooden pick inserted in centre of cupcake comes out clean. Let stand in pan for 10 minutes before removing to wire racks to cool completely.

Beat cream cheese and butter in large bowl until creamy. Add icing sugar and second amount of cocoa. Beat until smooth. Spoon into large resealable freezer bag with corner snipped off. Pipe onto cupcakes. Makes 12 cupcakes.

Pictured on page 143.

Tiramisu Angel Trifle

This decadent mocha-coloured dessert blends tiramisu flavours with a trifle method. If you have trouble finding coffee yogurt, purchase vanilla yogurt and stir in 2 tsp. (10 mL) of crushed instant coffee crystals.

Box of white angel food cake mix	15 oz.	430 g
Instant coffee granules, crushed to fine powder	2 tbsp.	30 mL
Box of instant vanilla pudding powder (6-serving size)	1	1
Milk	1 1/4 cups	300 mL
Coffee yogurt	4 cups	1 L
Frozen light whipped topping, thawed	4 cups	1 L
Cocoa, sifted if lumpy	1 tbsp.	15 mL

BEFORE: *1 cup (250 mL):*
540 Calories; *37.9 Total Fat (22.8 Sat); 254 mg Sodium*

AFTER: *1 cup (250 mL):*
255 Calories; *4.5 g Total Fat (0.5 g Mono, 0 g Poly, 4 g Sat); 6 mg Cholesterol; 50 g Carbohydrate; 0 g Fibre; 6 g Protein; 390 mg Sodium*

Combine cake mix and coffee granules in large bowl. Prepare cake mix according to package directions. Pour into ungreased 10 inch (25 cm) angel food tube pan with removable bottom. Spread evenly. Bake on bottom rack in 350°F (175°C) oven for about 45 minutes until top is browned, cracked and feels dry. Invert cake in pan onto glass bottle for 2 to 3 hours until cooled completely. Turn upright. Run knife around inside edge of pan to loosen cake. Remove bottom of pan with cake. Run knife around bottom and centre tube of pan to loosen cake. Cut half of cake into 1 inch (2.5 cm) cubes. Reserve remaining half for another use. Arrange half of cake cubes in 14 cup (3.5 L) trifle bowl or deep glass serving bowl.

Beat pudding powder and milk in medium bowl for 2 minutes. Add yogurt. Mix well. Spread half of yogurt mixture over cake.

Spread 2 cups whipped topping over yogurt mixture. Dust with 1 1/2 tsp. (7 mL) cocoa. Repeat layers with remaining cake cubes, yogurt mixture, whipped topping and cocoa. Chill, covered, for 4 hours. Makes about 12 cups (3 L).

Chocolate Turtles

Mmm...we just love this makeover of frozen chocolate turtle pie. After freezing, you can remove the chocolate turtles from the muffin cups and store in an airtight container in the freezer for up to two months.

Pretzel sticks, broken up	1 1/2 cups	375 mL
Liquid honey	1/4 cup	60 mL
Canola oil	2 tbsp.	30 mL
Skim milk	1/2 cup	125 mL
Cocoa, sifted if lumpy	1/4 cup	60 mL
Unsweetened chocolate baking squares (1 oz., 28 g, each), coarsely chopped	4	4
Non-fat vanilla yogurt	2 cups	500 mL
Can of low-fat sweetened condensed milk	11 oz.	300 mL
Chopped pecans, toasted (see Tip, page 110)	1/4 cup	60 mL

Put pretzels into large resealable freezer bag. Crush with rolling pin until coarse crumbs form. Transfer to small bowl. Add honey and canola oil. Stir well. Press into bottom of 12 greased muffin cups.

Whisk milk and cocoa in small saucepan until smooth. Add chocolate. Heat and stir on medium-low until chocolate is melted. Remove from heat.

Add yogurt and condensed milk. Whisk until smooth. Fill muffin cups.

Sprinkle with pecans. Freeze for at least 6 hours or overnight. Let stand for 10 minutes before serving. Makes 12 turtles.

BEFORE: *1 turtle: 375 Calories; 25 g Total Fat (11 g Sat); 206 mg Sodium*

AFTER: *1 turtle: 250 Calories; 10 g Total Fat (2.5 g Mono, 1 g Poly, 4 g Sat); 4 mg Cholesterol; 36 g Carbohydrate; 2 g Fibre; 7 g Protein; 185 mg Sodium*

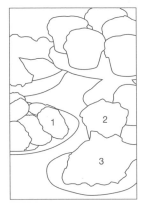

1. Chocolate Chip Cookies, page 139
2. Double Chocolate Cupcakes, page 140
3. Mango Peach Pie, page 138

Props: Casa Bugatti

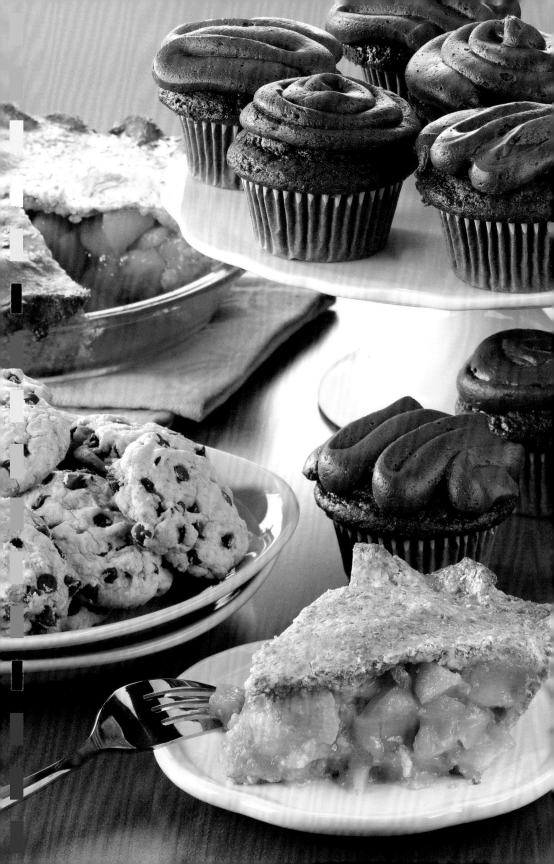

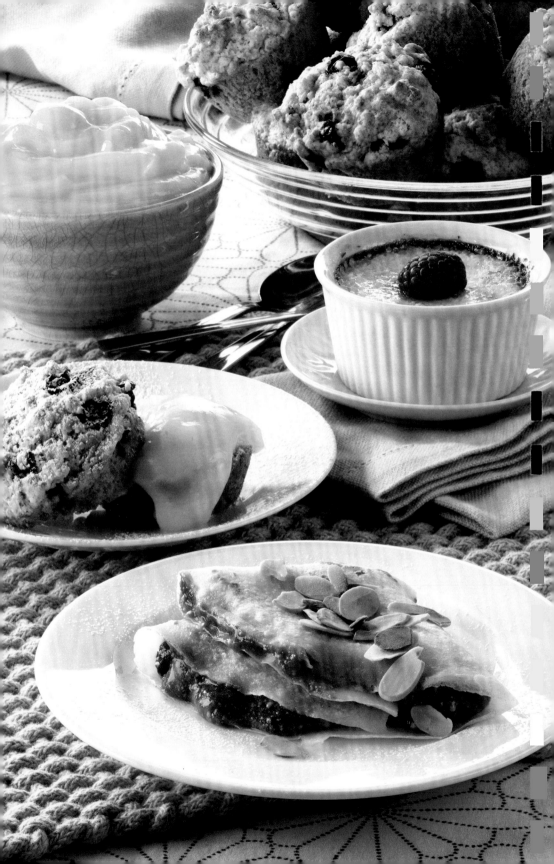

Lemon Coconut Crème Brûlée

Crème de la crème! The fresh lemon custard is truly superb, and the sugar and coconut crust gives this classic dessert an elegant finish.

Large eggs	3	3
Can of low-fat sweetened condensed milk	11 oz.	300 mL
Cornstarch	1 tbsp.	15 mL
Lemon juice	1 tbsp.	15 mL
Milk	1 1/2 cups	375 mL
Grated lemon zest (see Tip, page 151)	1 tbsp.	15 mL
Granulated sugar	2 tbsp.	30 mL
Medium unsweetened coconut	1 tbsp.	15 mL

Place six 6 oz. (170 mL) ramekins in ungreased 9 x 13 inch (23 x 33 cm) pan. Whisk first 4 ingredients in medium bowl.

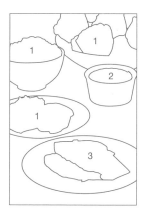

1. Cranberry Lemon Shortcakes, page 146
2. Lemon Coconut Crème Brûlée, above
3. Cherry Almond Crepes, page 148

Heat milk and lemon zest in small saucepan on medium until bubbles form around edge of saucepan. Remove from heat. Let stand, covered, for 10 minutes. Strain through fine sieve into small bowl. Slowly add milk mixture to egg mixture, whisking constantly. Pour into ramekins. Carefully pour boiling water into pan until halfway up sides of ramekins. Bake in 325°F (160°C) oven for about 35 minutes until custard is set along edges but centre still wobbles. Carefully remove ramekins from water. Place on wire rack to cool completely. Chill, covered, for at least 6 hours or overnight.

Process sugar and coconut in blender until finely ground. Sprinkle 1 1/2 tsp. (7 mL) over each ramekin. Broil on top rack in oven for about 4 minutes until browned and bubbling. Let stand for 5 minutes. Makes 6 crème brûlées.

Pictured at left.

BEFORE: *1 crème brulée: 362 Calories; 30 g Total Fat (**18 g Sat**); 35 mg Sodium*

AFTER: *1 crème brulée: 246 Calories; 5 g Total Fat (1 g Mono, 0 g Poly, **3 g Sat**); 80 mg Cholesterol; 38 g Carbohydrate; 0 g Fibre; 8 g Protein; 103 mg Sodium*

Cranberry Lemon Shortcakes

Tender scone-like biscuits are boosted with cranberries and filled with a light lemon cream.

All-purpose flour	1 cup	250 mL
Whole-wheat flour	1 cup	250 mL
Granulated sugar	1/3 cup	75 mL
Baking powder	1 tbsp.	15 mL
Baking soda	1/2 tsp.	2 mL
Salt	1/4 tsp.	1 mL
Cold butter	2 tbsp.	30 mL
Large egg	1	1
Skim milk	3/4 cup	175 mL
Canola oil	2 tbsp.	30 mL
Lemon juice	1 tbsp.	15 mL
Chopped fresh (or frozen, thawed) cranberries	1 cup	250 mL
Lemon spread	1 1/2 cups	375 mL
95% fat-free spreadable cream cheese	1/4 cup	60 mL
Lemon juice	1 tbsp.	15 mL
Grated lemon zest (see Tip, page 151)	1 tsp.	5 mL
Icing (confectioner's) sugar	1 tbsp.	15 mL

BEFORE: *1 shortcake:*
341 Calories; ***24 g Total Fat*** *(15 g Sat); 249 mg Sodium*

AFTER: *1 shortcake:*
220 Calories; ***6 g Total Fat*** *(2 g Mono, 1 g Poly, 2 g Sat); 19 mg Cholesterol; 38 g Carbohydrate; 2 g Fibre; 4 g Protein; 270 mg Sodium*

Combine first 6 ingredients in large bowl. Cut in butter until mixture resembles coarse crumbs.

Whisk next 4 ingredients in small bowl. Add to flour mixture. Add cranberries. Stir until just moistened. Spoon into 12 greased muffin cups. Bake in 400°F (205°C) oven for about 15 minutes until wooden pick inserted in centre comes out clean. Let stand in pan for 5 minutes before removing to wire racks to cool. Split biscuits in half horizontally. Place bottom halves on large serving plate.

Beat next 4 ingredients in medium bowl until smooth. Spoon over bottom halves of biscuits. Place top halves of biscuits over lemon mixture.

Dust with icing sugar. Makes 12 shortcakes.

Pictured on page 144.

Desserts

Banana Butterscotch Pie

Banana Cream Pie made over with a butterscotch twist! The versatile, lower-fat pastry cream can also be used as a filling for cake or other pies.

Graham cracker crumbs	1 1/4 cups	300 mL
Butter, melted	2 tbsp.	30 mL
Canola oil	2 tbsp.	30 mL
Granulated sugar	1 tbsp.	15 mL
Large egg	1	1
Cornstarch	2 tbsp.	30 mL
All-purpose flour	1 tbsp.	15 mL
Skim milk	1 1/3 cups	325 mL
Butterscotch ice cream topping	1/2 cup	125 mL
Sliced banana	2 cups	500 mL
Frozen light whipped topping, thawed	1 cup	250 mL

BEFORE: *1 wedge:*
662 Calories; *45 g Total Fat (27.2 g Sat); 407 mg Sodium*

AFTER: *1 wedge:*
260 Calories; *9 g Total Fat (3 g Mono, 1 g Poly, 3 g Sat); 26 mg Cholesterol; 43 g Carbohydrate; 2 g Fibre; 3 g Protein; 219 mg Sodium*

Combine first 4 ingredients in medium bowl. Press firmly in bottom and up side of greased 9 inch (23 cm) pie plate. Bake in 350°F (175°C) oven for 10 minutes. Let stand on wire rack until cool.

Whisk next 3 ingredients in small saucepan. Slowly add milk, whisking constantly. Add ice cream topping. Cook on medium for about 10 minutes, stirring constantly, until mixture is bubbling and thickened.

Arrange 1 cup (250 mL) banana slices over crust. Pour butterscotch mixture over banana. Smooth top. Chill for about 2 hours until set. Cover with remaining banana slices.

Spread whipped topping over banana. Cuts into 8 wedges.

Cherry Almond Crepes

These delicate crepes can be kept at room temperature for a few hours until you're ready to serve them, or made up to one day ahead and kept in the refrigerator. To reheat, stack crepes on a baking sheet or ovenproof platter and cover with foil, then place in a 200°F (95°C) oven for about one hour.

ALMOND CREPES

All-purpose flour	1 cup	250 mL
Ground almonds	1/2 cup	125 mL
Granulated sugar	2 tbsp.	30 mL
Salt	1/2 tsp.	2 mL
Egg whites (large)	3	3
Skim milk	1 1/3 cups	325 mL
Canola oil	2 tbsp.	30 mL
Almond extract	1/2 tsp.	2 mL

CHERRY RICOTTA FILLING

Can of cherry pie filling	19 oz.	540 mL
Light ricotta cheese	1/2 cup	125 mL
Lemon juice	2 tsp.	10 mL
Icing (confectioner's) sugar	1 tbsp.	15 mL
Sliced almonds, toasted (see Tip, page 110)	1/4 cup	60 mL

BEFORE: *1 stuffed crepe: 350 Calories; **22 g Total Fat** (11 g Sat); 227 mg Sodium*

AFTER: *1 stuffed crepe: 230 Calories; **8 g Total Fat** (4.5 g Mono, 2 g Poly, 1 g Sat); 5 mg Cholesterol; 34 g Carbohydrate; 2 g Fibre; 7 g Protein; 177 mg Sodium*

Almond Crepes: Combine first 4 ingredients in large bowl. Make a well in centre.

Add next 4 ingredients to well. Whisk until smooth. Let stand for 30 minutes. Heat small (8 inch, 20 cm) non-stick frying pan on medium. Spray with cooking spray. Stir batter. Pour 1/4 cup (60 mL) batter into pan. Immediately swirl to coat bottom, lifting and tilting pan to ensure entire bottom is covered. Cook for about 1 minute until top is set and brown spots appear on bottom. Turn crepe over. Cook until brown spots appear on bottom. Remove to plate. Cover to keep warm. Repeat with remaining batter, stirring batter each time to distribute almonds, and spraying pan with cooking spray if necessary to prevent sticking. Makes about 10 crepes.

(continued on next page)

Cherry Ricotta Filling: Stir first 3 ingredients in medium bowl. Makes about 2 3/4 cups (675 mL). Spoon filling onto crepes. Fold crepes into quarters. Arrange on platter.

Dust with icing sugar. Sprinkle with almonds. Makes about 10 stuffed crepes.

Pictured on page 144.

Super Fruit Pizza

A great make-ahead dessert that is sure to impress your guests. Rolled oats in the crust add fibre. Any fruit can be used for the toppings, but we've opted for a trio of berries, which are superfoods!

95% fat-free spreadable cream cheese	1 cup	250 mL
Granulated sugar	1/4 cup	60 mL
Vanilla extract	1/2 tsp.	2 mL
All-purpose flour	1 1/4 cups	300 mL
Quick-cooking rolled oats	1 cup	250 mL
Granulated sugar	1/3 cup	75 mL
Butter, melted	1/4 cup	60 mL
Canola oil	3 tbsp.	50 mL
Fresh (or frozen, thawed) blueberries	1 1/2 cups	375 mL
Fresh (or frozen, thawed) raspberries	1 cup	250 mL
Sliced fresh strawberries	1 cup	250 mL
Sliced almonds, toasted (see Tip, page 110)	1/4 cup	60 mL

BEFORE: *1 wedge:*
239 Calories; 17 g Total Fat
(8 g Sat)*; 100 mg Sodium*

AFTER: *1 wedge:*
170 Calories; 7 g Total Fat
(3 g Mono, 1 g Poly,
2.5 g Sat*);*
13 mg Cholesterol;
23 g Carbohydrate;
2 g Fibre; 4 g Protein;
120 mg Sodium

Beat first 3 ingredients in small bowl until smooth. Chill, covered, until ready to use.

Combine next 5 ingredients in medium bowl until mixture resembles coarse crumbs. Press evenly into greased 12 inch (30 cm) pizza pan. Bake in 350°F (175°C) oven for about 15 minutes until golden. Let stand on wire rack until cool. Spread cream cheese mixture over crust, almost to edge.

Arrange next 3 ingredients over top. Sprinkle with almonds. Cuts into 16 wedges.

Key Lime Dessert

You're thinking, "Tofu in a dessert? Are they crazy?" No—just trust us and try it! The silky, creamy lime topping goes very nicely with the light graham crumb crust.

Graham cracker crumbs	1 1/3 cups	325 mL
Butter, melted	2 tbsp.	30 mL
Canola oil	2 tbsp.	30 mL
Granulated sugar	1 tbsp.	15 mL
Firm light silken tofu, well drained	12 oz.	340 g
Can of low-fat sweetened condensed milk	11 oz.	300 mL
Block light cream cheese, softened	4 oz.	125 g
Lime juice	1/2 cup	125 mL
Grated lime zest (see Tip, page 151)	1 tsp.	5 mL

BEFORE: *1 square:*
224 Calories; **15 g Total Fat** *(9 g Sat); 198 mg Sodium*

AFTER: *1 square:*
150 Calories; **6 g Total Fat** *(1.5 g Mono, 0.5 g Poly, 2 g Sat); 10 mg Cholesterol; 19 g Carbohydrate; 0 g Fibre; 4 g Protein; 143 mg Sodium*

Combine first 4 ingredients in medium bowl. Press firmly into greased 9 x 9 inch (23 x 23 cm) pan. Bake in 325°F (160°C) oven for 10 minutes. Let stand on wire rack until cool.

Process remaining 5 ingredients in blender or food processor, scraping down sides if necessary, until smooth. Spread evenly over crust. Chill for at least 6 hours or overnight until set. Cuts into 16 squares.

Mocha Layer Cake

A decadent, old-fashioned–looking layer cake with a fraction of the fat. Less than 300 calories for a great big piece! It's so easy to throw together that it'll become your go-to cake for special occasions—or just because.

All-purpose flour	1 3/4 cups	425 mL
Granulated sugar	1 cup	250 mL
Baking soda	1 tsp.	5 mL
Salt	1/2 tsp.	2 mL
Hot strong prepared coffee	1 cup	250 mL
Cocoa, sifted if lumpy	1/2 cup	125 mL

(continued on next page)

1% buttermilk	1/2 cup	125 mL
Egg whites (about 2 large)	1/4 cup	60 mL
Vanilla extract	1 tsp.	5 mL

FLUFFY MOCHA FROSTING

Cold strong prepared coffee	1 cup	250 mL
Box of instant fat-free chocolate pudding powder (4-serving size)	1	1
Frozen 95% fat-free whipped topping, thawed	3 cups	750 mL

BEFORE: *1 wedge:*
970 Calories; 65 g Total Fat (34 g Sat); 592 mg Sodium

AFTER: *1 wedge:*
280 Calories; 2.5 g Total Fat (0.5 g Mono, 0 g Poly, 1 g Sat); 5 mg Cholesterol; 60 g Carbohydrate; 3 g Fibre; 6 g Protein; 490 mg Sodium

Line bottom of two 8 inch (20 cm) round pans with parchment paper circles. Spray sides with cooking spray. Set aside. Combine first 4 ingredients in large bowl.

Whisk first amount of coffee and cocoa in small bowl until cocoa is dissolved.

Combine next 3 ingredients in medium bowl. Stir in coffee mixture. Add to flour mixture. Stir until just combined. Spread evenly in prepared pans. Bake in 350°F (175°C) oven for about 20 minutes until wooden pick inserted in centre of cake comes out clean. Let stand in pans for 10 minutes before inverting onto wire racks to cool completely. Cut each cake in half horizontally to make 4 layers.

Fluffy Mocha Frosting: Beat second amount of coffee and pudding powder in medium bowl for 2 minutes. Add 1 cup (250 mL) whipped topping. Stir until combined. Fold in remaining whipped topping. Makes about 3 1/4 cups (800 mL). Chill for 30 minutes. Place 1 cake layer on serving plate. Spread with about 1/2 cup (125 mL) frosting. Repeat with second and third cake layers, spreading about 1/2 cup (125 mL) frosting between each layer. Cover with remaining cake layer. Spread remaining frosting over top and sides of cake. Chill for at least 1 hour. Cuts into 8 wedges.

Pictured on front cover.

 tip When a recipe calls for grated zest and juice, it's easier to grate the fruit first, then juice it. Be careful not to grate down to the pith (white part of the peel), which is bitter and best avoided.

Almond Fruit-Trio Crisp

Gluten-free

An inviting combination of plums, apples and pears is topped with a lower-fat, gluten-free crumb topping. Very comforting.

Brown sugar, packed	1/2 cup	125 mL
Apple juice	1/4 cup	60 mL
Cornstarch	2 tbsp.	30 mL
Ground cinnamon	1 tsp.	5 mL
Ground allspice	1/4 tsp.	1 mL
Sliced black (or red) plums	2 cups	500 mL
Sliced peeled cooking apple (such as McIntosh)	2 cups	500 mL
Sliced peeled pear	2 cups	500 mL
Ground almonds	1 cup	250 mL
Medium sweetened coconut	2/3 cup	150 mL
Brown sugar, packed	1/4 cup	60 mL
Butter, melted	2 tbsp.	30 mL
Canola oil	2 tbsp.	30 mL
Sliced natural almonds	1/4 cup	60 mL

BEFORE: *1/2 cup (125 mL):*
401 calories; *17.8 Total Fat (6.5 g Sat); 178 mg Sodium*

AFTER: *1/2 cup (125 mL):*
216 Calories; *11 g Total Fat (5 g Mono, 2 g Poly, 3.5 g Sat); 5 mg Cholesterol; 28 g Carbohydrate; 3 g Fibre; 3 g Protein; 35 mg Sodium*

Combine first 5 ingredients in large bowl. Add next 3 ingredients. Stir. Transfer to greased 2 quart (2 L) casserole.

Combine next 5 ingredients in small bowl until mixture resembles coarse crumbs. Scatter over fruit mixture.

Sprinkle with sliced almonds. Bake, uncovered, in 375°F (190°C) oven for about 35 minutes until apple is tender and topping is golden. Makes about 6 cups (1.5 L).

Paré Pointer

He's not too short and not too tall. He's Fahrenheit.

Ginger Cheesecake

Cheesecake is a time-honoured indulgence, but you definitely don't need to feel bad about enjoying a slice of this dessert every now and then! The creamy ginger filling is much lower in fat than usual cheesecakes.

CRUST		
Quick-cooking rolled oats	1 cup	250 mL
All-purpose flour	1/3 cup	75 mL
Canola oil	1/4 cup	60 mL
Finely chopped pecans, toasted (see Tip, page 110)	1/4 cup	60 mL
Brown sugar, packed	2 tbsp.	30 mL
FILLING		
Light ricotta cheese	2 cups	500 mL
Block light cream cheese, cut up and softened	8 oz.	250 g
Brown sugar, packed	1/2 cup	125 mL
Ginger marmalade	1/2 cup	125 mL
All-purpose flour	2 tbsp.	30 mL
Salt	1/8 tsp.	0.5 mL
Egg whites (large)	2	2
Large eggs	2	2
Minced crystallized ginger	1/3 cup	75 mL

BEFORE: *1 wedge:*
512 Calories; *39 g Total Fat (21.6 Sat); 471 mg Sodium*

AFTER: *1 wedge:*
305 Calories; *14 g Total Fat (5 g Mono, 2 g Poly, 5 g Sat); 48 mg Cholesterol; 36 g Carbohydrate; 1 g Fibre; 9 g Protein; 194 mg Sodium*

Crust: Combine all 5 ingredients in medium bowl until mixture resembles coarse crumbs. Press firmly into bottom of greased 9 inch (23 cm) springform pan. Bake in 350°F (175°C) oven for about 15 minutes until edges just turn golden. Let stand on wire rack to cool.

Filling: Beat first 6 ingredients in large bowl until smooth.

Add egg whites. Beat until just combined. Add eggs, 1 at a time, beating after each addition until just combined.

Stir in ginger. Spread evenly over crust. Bake in 350°F (175°C) oven for about 65 minutes until puffed along edges but centre still wobbles. Immediately run knife around inside edge of pan to allow cheesecake to settle evenly. Let stand on wire rack to cool completely. Chill, covered, for at least 6 hours or overnight. Cuts into 12 wedges.

Measurement Tables

Throughout this book measurements are given in Conventional and Metric measure. To compensate for differences between the two measurements due to rounding, a full metric measure is not always used. The cup used is the standard 8 fluid ounce. Temperature is given in degrees Fahrenheit and Celsius. Baking pan measurements are in inches and centimetres as well as quarts and litres. An exact metric conversion is given below as well as the working equivalent (Metric Standard Measure).

Spoons

Conventional Measure	Metric Exact Conversion Millilitre (mL)	Metric Standard Measure Millilitre (mL)
1/8 teaspoon (tsp.)	0.6 mL	0.5 mL
1/4 teaspoon (tsp.)	1.2 mL	1 mL
1/2 teaspoon (tsp.)	2.4 mL	2 mL
1 teaspoon (tsp.)	4.7 mL	5 mL
2 teaspoons (tsp.)	9.4 mL	10 mL
1 tablespoon (tbsp.)	14.2 mL	15 mL

Cups

Conventional Measure	Metric Exact Conversion Millilitre (mL)	Metric Standard Measure Millilitre (mL)
1/4 cup (4 tbsp.)	56.8 mL	60 mL
1/3 cup (5 1/3 tbsp.)	75.6 mL	75 mL
1/2 cup (8 tbsp.)	113.7 mL	125 mL
2/3 cup (10 2/3 tbsp.)	151.2 mL	150 mL
3/4 cup (12 tbsp.)	170.5 mL	175 mL
1 cup (16 tbsp.)	227.3 mL	250 mL
4 1/2 cups	1022.9 mL	1000 mL (1 L)

Oven Temperatures

Fahrenheit (°F)	Celsius (°C)
175°	80°
200°	95°
225°	110°
250°	120°
275°	140°
300°	150°
325°	160°
350°	175°
375°	190°
400°	205°
425°	220°
450°	230°
475°	240°
500°	260°

Dry Measurements

Conventional Measure Ounces (oz.)	Metric Exact Conversion Grams (g)	Metric Standard Measure Grams (g)
1 oz.	28.3 g	28 g
2 oz.	56.7 g	57 g
3 oz.	85.0 g	85 g
4 oz.	113.4 g	125 g
5 oz.	141.7 g	140 g
6 oz.	170.1 g	170 g
7 oz.	198.4 g	200 g
8 oz.	226.8 g	250 g
16 oz.	453.6 g	500 g
32 oz.	907.2 g	1000 g (1 kg)

Pans

Conventional Inches	Metric Centimetres
8x8 inch	20x20 cm
9x9 inch	23x23 cm
9x13 inch	23x33 cm
10x15 inch	25x38 cm
11x17 inch	28x43 cm
8x2 inch round	20x5 cm
9x2 inch round	23x5 cm
10x4 1/2 inch tube	25x11 cm
8x4x3 inch loaf	20x10x7.5 cm
9x5x3 inch loaf	23x12.5x7.5 cm

Casseroles

CANADA & BRITAIN Standard Size Casserole	Exact Metric Measure	UNITED STATES Standard Size Casserole	Exact Metric Measure
1 qt. (5 cups)	1.13 L	1 qt. (4 cups)	900 mL
1 1/2 qts. (7 1/2 cups)	1.69 L	1 1/2 qts. (6 cups)	1.35 L
2 qts. (10 cups)	2.25 L	2 qts. (8 cups)	1.8 L
2 1/2 qts. (12 1/2 cups)	2.81 L	2 1/2 qts. (10 cups)	2.25 L
3 qts. (15 cups)	3.38 L	3 qts. (12 cups)	2.7 L
4 qts. (20 cups)	4.5 L	4 qts. (16 cups)	3.6 L
5 qts. (25 cups)	5.63 L	5 qts. (20 cups)	4.5 L

Recipe Index

Low Sodium

M

N

O

P

Q

R

S